HUMAN RESOURCES
IN HEALTH CARE

HUMAN RESOURCES IN HEALTH CARE
A MANAGER'S GUIDE

Anthony J. Strike
MIPD, DMS, Cert. Ed

**Blackwell
Science**

© 1995 by Anthony J. Strike
Blackwell Science Ltd
Editorial Offices:
Osney Mead, Oxford OX2 0EL
25 John Street, London WC1N 2BL
23 Ainslie Place, Edinburgh EH3 6AJ
238 Main Street, Cambridge
  Massachusetts 02142, USA
54 University Street, Carlton
  Victoria 3053, Australia

Other Editorial Offices:
  Arnette Blackwell SA
  1, rue de Lille, 75007 Paris
  France

Blackwell Wissenshafts-Verlag GmbH
Kurfürstendamm 57
10707 Berlin, Germany

Feldgasse 13, A-1238 Wien
Austria

First published 1995

Set in 10/13 Melior
by DP Photosetting, Aylesbury, Bucks
Printed and bound in Great Britain
by Hartnolls Ltd, Bodmin, Cornwall.

DISTRIBUTORS

Marston Book Services Ltd
PO Box 87
Oxford OX2 0DT
(*Orders:* Tel: 01865 791155
        Fax: 01865 791927
        Telex: 837515)

USA
Blackwell Science, Inc.
238 Main Street
Cambridge, MA 02142
(*Orders:* Tel: 800 215-1000
                617 876-7000
           Fax: 617 492-5263)

Canada
Oxford University Press
70 Wynford Drive
Don Mills
Ontario M3C 1J9
(*Orders:* Tel: 416 441 2941)

Australia
Blackwell Science Pty Ltd
54 University Street
Carlton, Victoria 3053
(*Orders:* Tel: 03 347-0300
           Fax: 03 349-3016)

A catalogue record for this title
is available from the British Library

ISBN 0–632–03974–4

Library of Congress
Cataloging-in-Publication Data
is available

CONTENTS

The author of this book is a rare bird – a specialist prepared to give away his secrets. Not only is Anthony Strike prepared to accept that the skills he has assembled over the years can be better exercised by other people but he is also prepared to put himself out to ensure that those taking on these responsibilities are best equipped to use them. His sense of the need to do this derives from a deep understanding of how the National Health Service has changed since the reforms of 1991 and in particular how these changes have affected the personnel function. Unlike those who have tried to cling on to their traditional power bases, the author has risen to the challenge of finding new ways of exercising his influence.

This book is not an academic treatise, the logic of the positions set out in the various chapters is compelling and carries intellectual conviction. Taken together with the author's clarity of style and ear for a telling phrase, this ensures that the book is an easy as well as an authoritative read. It eschews jargon and the definitions offered of terms which are bandied around the NHS with evident lack of understanding are immensely helpful. The exercises which are set put these definitions in a practical context in a manner which fixes their meaning firmly in the readers' minds. NHS personnel managers have in the past suffered from the fact that everybody thinks they know about 'personnel'. Has anybody ever encountered a manager who thinks he or she is poor at managing his or her staff? But turn the question on its head and ask staff what they think about how well they are managed and the answer is, more often than not, a resounding No. This book essentially takes that position as its starting point and attempts to tackle these particular forms of self-delusion by offering practical advice and guidance.

Though every chapter of the book makes absorbing reading, some chapters warrant special attention. I have in mind the chapters on Human Resources Planning, Labour Utilization,

Reward and Performance. All these focus on areas where real improvements are needed and where a great deal of under-standing and skill needs to be acquired in a short time. In all these areas the book offers practical approaches. There is no point in the book where what is proposed is less than clear. There is no need for head scratching and nobody needs to call for wet towels.

Most of all, the book is a modern book. It is up-to-date and contains the very latest applied thinking. It deals with the NHS as it is today – not as it was nor as it might be. For all these reasons it deserves not only to be read but to be used.

PREFACE

It is my clear hope in writing this book that in receiving, borrowing or purchasing a copy you will see in the words a reflection of your own practice. If successful in the first aim, of writing a real and practical account, my second aim is to enable you to turn the words that follow into action.

I sincerely hope I have achieved both of my aims and that what you gain from this book more than compensates for the price on its cover and for your time invested in reading it.

In some parts of the text management practice is considered within areas of employment which are the subject of statutory duties or requirements. While I have made every attempt to provide for accuracy, this book should not be taken as a guide to the law.

This book does represent a freeze-frame of a thinking process. It is sad that it has to be frozen in time, as the learning process it represents is continuous. I hope you will, in assimilating the content of the book, find it a stimulus to developing your own thoughts.

Anthony J. Strike
June 1995

ACKNOWLEDGEMENTS

Portsmouth Hospitals NHS Trust, my current employers, have provided me with a rich source of experience reflected in this book. The views expressed in the text which follows are my own and not necessarily the views or policies of Portsmouth Hospitals NHS Trust Board nor those of the panel of reviewers.

The panel of people listed below commented on the manuscript, and the final product is much richer as a result of their time and attention. Thanks are due to:

> Mr T. Plant, Pay Strategy and Research Manager, Anglia and Oxford Regional Health Authority.
> Mr W. Barnott, Personnel Manager, Portsmouth Healthcare NHS Trust.
> Mrs S. Smart, Directorate General Manager, Portsmouth Hospitals NHS Trust.
> Mr B. MacKenzie, Senior Lecturer, Centre for Care, Independent and Public Sector Management, University of Portsmouth.
> Mr S. Pimbblet, Personnel Manager, Bowman Distribution Europe (UK) Limited.

The manuscript was prepared and repeatedly amended by Miss Ilsa Dalmut to whom I am grateful for both her efficiency and patience.

The last words of acknowledgement go to my wife, Caroline, who was to raise our daughter for nine months while I gave birth to this book! Neither would have been possible without her constant support.

Chapter 1:
INTRODUCING HEALTH
SERVICE HUMAN
RESOURCE MANAGEMENT

Introduction

The purpose of this first chapter is to set a context or back cloth for the rest of the book. It will examine health services, their reform and complexity. The distinction between management and personnel management is considered with the impact of the changing environment upon them. This chapter sets out the rationale for the book and the assumptions made in writing it.

Learning outcomes

- To understand the economic pressures on health services and the effect of those pressures on management and personnel management.

- To perceive the distinction between management of staff as a line manager and personnel management as a professional function.

- To understand the current policies and structures within the National Health Service (NHS).

- To see the personnel management agenda that the above economic pressures and current policies produce as their natural consequence.

Scanning the environment

The content of health care human resource management in the 1990s

The health service of the 1990s is not that of the 1980s. Change in public and political organizations is perhaps inevitable.

Managers in the contemporary health service have seen something of a revolution take place; some revolutions are bloodless but this one was in parts bloody. Survivor managers took the final leap from 1980s administrators to 1990s executives. Many of the former centralized controls have gone and decision-making increasingly lies in the hands of local managers of services. The functional specialisms of health service management are at the same time giving way to true general management. These changes have challenged managers to learn, survive and thrive within a new environment.

Wider political and organizational changes which introduced the internal market and competition for care provision have promoted a new financial and business orientated culture. The health service is now dominated by self-governing NHS Trusts which have the legal status to employ staff in the numbers and on the terms they think appropriate. This major delegated power gives managers in NHS Trusts control over some 75% of their annual recurring costs. The health service is labour intensive and managers in NHS Trusts, as distinct employers, have complete responsibility for those staff. Effective staff management is essential to ensure services thrive in an increasingly competitive market of private and public care providers.

Despite continually falling waiting times the numbers on waiting lists still suggest that demand for health care will not plateau and the ability or willingness of the nation to pay will certainly not match demand. Health care in principle, but not in reality, is still free at the point of delivery in the United Kingdom.

Health provision is not by any means free. People do pay for health care – mainly through national insurance and general taxation, but also through private health insurance in anticipation of requiring the services later. In the public sphere the clear disconnection between use and payment means that people expect unlimited provision to meet their clinical or social needs and expectations, but with a minimal effect on their pockets. Governments and insurance companies have to walk the line between acceptable levels of taxation or premiums and their spending requirements. Health services have to make the best use of the money they receive. If maximum benefit is not obtained from every pound the equation shifts against further investment. To get the most out of each extra pound sterling it has to be used for the achievement of health gain. This is where the new health 'Purchasers' have a part to play. Purchasers act on behalf of the paying public. If patients paid directly for care then clinical rationing would not exist. Ability and willingness to pay would replace clinical rationing of care provision, clinical rationing being based on meeting need rather than want or demand as expressed by ability to pay.

Public health services are not now entirely free at the point of delivery: direct charges are made for prescriptions, dental services, ophthalmic services and appliances, and for ambulances used at road traffic accidents. The recent reforms increasingly link cash to work on a cost-per-case basis, but without that necessarily being a charge directly to the individual patient.

The changing face of personnel management

The increasing demand for effective health care purchasing, i.e. a more intelligent and discriminating purchaser, requires a more discriminating provider. Health care providers need to be better able to control the health care offered rather than providing what their clinicians internally believe is of interest or appropriate.

Personnel management as a profession and a discipline has also altered. With a change in the wider national industrial relations scene, associated legislative change and falling union membership, and with an accompanying national recession, private sector managers have had to fight for survival and have needed to restructure their organizations' labour forces to help ensure that survival. Nationally, across all industry sectors, personnel managers have worried less about good labour relations and more about the value of labour as an organizational resource. Whether this change of emphasis was prompted by or was simply not prevented by the statutory regulation of the trade unions is a matter of interpretation. To this end personnel management ceased to be the judge of fairness and equity, no longer the ethical heart of the organization but rather instrumental to its commercial or business success. These changes to the personnel function are explored further in Chapter 9.

Within the health service also, service managers must take hold of this new human resource management agenda for staff in their own span of control. Leaving the administration of staff management to personnel support specialists may be sustainable but working within the strategic human resources agenda for the organization to which any manager belongs is essential. Abdicating responsibility for managing the most expensive and essential element of any health service to third party specialists is not the behaviour of entrepreneurial managers who intend to see their service succeed. Likert (1967) stated that 'of all the tasks of management, managing the human component is the central and most important task, because all else depends on how well it is done'.

The new management agenda

Why is it important for managers to grasp this described agenda? A fundamental shift in the focus of responsibility has taken place in health services. The focus of provision has moved from District Health Authorities to self-governing NHS Trusts. Social services, general practitioners, voluntary and private organizations have a presence but illness as a business is dominated by NHS Trusts. The realities of the internal market are such that local human resource management is not optional if services are to be successful. Contestability and competition now exists. The last 40 years' accumulation of national regulations about staff management simply cannot survive the new competitive pressures. The new dynamic health care environment requires a pace of change which in turn demands a flexible staff resource. Managers cannot afford to fight a 'personnel bureaucracy'.

Why this book?

This book is not an academic account or interpretation, but an account of the current realities of working inside the health service as a manager of staff. It is not a text on personnel management; many already exist although they are not usually specific to health services. Nor is this book a study of health services in the abstract. It is about the practical management of staff in health services, highlighting the personnel agenda for managers specific to their organizational context. Personnel management as a specialist discipline is distinct and separate from the line management of staff undertaken by managers. This book is concerned with the latter activity. It tries to address the advantages, challenges and dilemmas for managers employed within the health care sector so that new ideas and techniques can be directly applied within local and unique surroundings. This book is not written as an aid in supervisory skills or in managing individual staff but offers practical guidance on the wider staff management agenda. Being a practical text it is not necessary that managers read it cover to cover. Each chapter has been written as a self contained unit which can be read independently of the others.

The task

Managing a diverse workforce

The NHS across the UK employs over one million people. In broad terms staff can be classified into the following types:

- medical,
- dental,
- nursing,
- midwifery,
- professions allied to medicine,
- technical,
- scientific,
- ancillary,
- maintenance,
- administrative,
- works,
- ambulance, and
- management.

While this may seem a long list of possibilities, each contains a sub-classification of specialisms and trades, for example professional staff allied to medicine include:

- chiropodists,
- dietitians,
- occupational therapists,
- orthoptists,
- physiotherapists,
- radiographers,
- pharmacists, and
- speech therapists.

Within each profession a career structure exists, for example:

- Helper,
- Physiotherapist,
- Senior II Physiotherapist,
- Senior I Physiotherapist,
- Superintendent Physiotherapist, and so on.

It is quickly realized that health services represent a very large and complex human organization. Health services employ many people with a great range of experience, skills and talents. Managers may come from any one of the health care professions, or from none, and do not and cannot understand them all. Managing health services effectively is a complex but not impossible task. Managers do survive and cope with the complexity. Johnson and Scholes (1988) state:

> 'In practice managers cope with the range of influences by evolving, over time, accepted wisdom about their industry, its environment and what are sensible responses to different situations.'

What is meant by management?

Any person who is accountable for a resource, whether it be staff, money, buildings or land, is a manager of that resource. A ward manager (or sister) has considerable resources to command. The service, directorate, specialty or locality managers to whom first-line managers (like ward managers) report can account for anything from 50 to 1 000 staff and so at that level managing personnel becomes a significant part of their role. These managers may well have either a personnel manager accountable to them or a named contact point in a central personnel department for support purposes.

What is meant by 'personnel'?

In the health service personnel departments are increasingly becoming more streamlined and their functions and responsibilities are being devolved to line managers. Many managers are familiar with (and indeed may take for granted) responsibility for day to day tasks like:

- job advertising,
- selection interviewing,
- induction,
- appraisal,
- development,
- staff grievances,
- discipline, and
- sanctions.

These are in many cases seen as essential management tasks which cannot and should not be left to a third party personnel manager. These, it may be argued, are not the areas of personnel management which have maximum impact on organizational success. The day-to-day issues listed above are the areas which, if devolved, release numbers of specialist personnel staff and allow savings. More recently service and general managers, especially in clinical directorate or locality structures, have either had areas of personnel responsibility devolved to them or have actively sought control of areas of personnel policy. This is entirely sensible given the managers' accountability for the future success of the services they manage and which provide employment. It is this new agenda the book addresses.

Some managers may decide the scope or content of this book reaches beyond their current freedom to act. If so, the ideas should act as a spur to thought about why this is so and whether their current role restrictions are productive or bureaucratic.

Throughout this book the text is interrupted by short exercises or activities aimed at setting the manager in the direction suggested or to make a particular part of the text specific to the local context. Each is headed 'Activity' as shown below.

Activity

Make or obtain a list of the numbers and different types of staff you manage within your team, the grades you employ within each and the numbers involved. Consider the complexity of this situation.

In addition state alongside each line in your list a specific task undertaken by each different staff type which differentiates them from the others.

New policies

Certain policies are being pursued in the health sector, if not the public sector, which manifest themselves in structure. These policies are broadly as follows.

Consumerism

Encouraging the public as individuals, rather than as a collectivity, to demand access, quality and choice from health services; so creating competition.

Devolution

> Passing decision-making and responsibility closer to the individual patient and controlling what happens through contracts, standards or agreements concerning outcomes.

Outplacement

> Developing the range of choices open to individual consumers by accepting that an internal competitive monopoly in care provision by NHS Trusts is not necessarily desirable.

Minimalism

> Expecting health services to deliver ever increasing levels of care from a limited if not shrinking level of available resources.

Management

> Running the health service like a business, with economic and financial considerations having equal if not greater value in ensuring survival than professional or clinical standards.

What has changed

The specific structural changes which reflect the above policies are characterized by:

- District Health Authorities (through the contracting process) becoming purchasers of NHS care provision rather than administrators of it;
- directly managed units, as care providers, competing for contracts from purchasers;
- directly managed units (through application) becoming self-governing NHS Trusts and free of District Health Authority management;
- the merger of District Health Authorities and Family Health Service Authorities to form new Unitary Purchasing Commissions;
- general practitioners making applications to become fund-holding (and so able to purchase care directly, rather than through their District Health Authority);
- Regional Health Authorities in England being abolished; and
- eight NHS Executive Regional Offices being created as an extension of the civil service to manage the market.

The structure of health services

The key bodies in the Health Service now are as illustrated in Figure 1.1.

The NHS executive

This ensures public accountability for the paying public by regulating the market and ensuring national health policies are implemented.

Purchasing authorities or commissions

Following an assessment of the health needs of their resident population these authorities purchase large volumes of care for residents in their geographic area from the source providing best quality and value.

Self-governing trusts

These, on securing contracts for the provision of care, act to meet those contracts in delivering health care services while meeting certain statutory duties.

Fundholding general practitioners

These can provide care directly to their population in the primary care setting and are increasingly choosing to do so; and

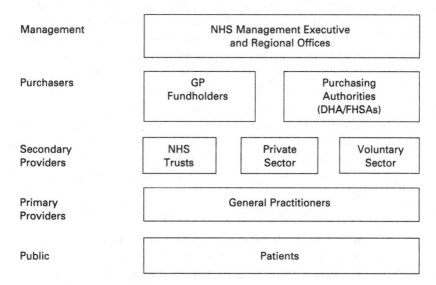

Figure 1.1 Health service structure.

they can also purchase additional secondary care, either directly or by influencing the main purchaser.

This structure maximizes the potential for a variety of providers to be introduced into the health care market, to allow choices between those providers and so promote competition. While NHS Trusts remain state institutions which dominate the health market this situation may potentially change. A new set of core values is emerging within the health service around efficiency, effectiveness, easy access, guaranteed standards, responsiveness and choice. Historical notions of equity, need, standardization, public service and public provision are being challenged.

Self-governing NHS Trusts

By introducing the legal concept of an NHS Trust, the government gave local managers control and ownership of local health resources. As separate legal bodies Trusts employ staff as employers in their own right and so are free to offer unique terms and pay. Trusts also have to raise sufficient income to meet their cost bases (including capital costs) by providing services, and so must enter into contracts. This revenue may come from working for Commissions, the main purchasers, or fundholding general practitioners, private patients or indeed by providing non-clinical services to external organizations.

To gain revenue Trusts must price their services (for sale) and those prices must both reflect true costs and be competitive. To meet one of their statutory duties prices need to cover all of the Trust's costs, including depreciation of assets, plus a 6% return on assets. Failing to set accurately the real price of services may mean gaining contracts for work but operating at a loss. One service cannot cross-subsidize another but each must compete on its own merits. Trusts cannot seek to make more than a 6% return on NHS work but can maximize profit from the private sector.

The statutory or required duties placed on Trusts are to:

- break even, taking one year with another,
- achieve a minimum return of 6% on assets,
- stay within their external financing limit,
- publish five year strategic directions,

- produce annual business plans,
- publish an annual report and accounts,
- hold at least one annual public meeting, and
- gain contracts from purchasers for care provision.

In theory, if increasingly not in practice, if Trusts have no contract to provide care then they cannot provide it. If care is provided over and above or without a contract covering that activity then it may not be paid for. Hospitals or services without work do not receive income and so have to reduce their capacity and costs. Successful hospitals or services have resources to invest. Two ideas hold sway: that money follows patients and that competition between Trusts improves the options available to those patients. Money is not allocated to budgets against a formula as was previously the case.

Choices between competing trusts

Instead of hospitals or services looking to regulate activity (by putting patients or clients on lists) in order to control their expenditure against allocated budgets, now services need patient activity to create those budgets. The purchasers, in making choices between providers, are sensitive to:

- price,
- quality of care,
- waiting times,
- location,
- access,
- standards of accommodation,
- contract monitoring information, and
- government health policy.

Impact on personnel matters

The staff management agenda is influenced both by what is happening to health services and by wider employment issues. These include:

- the legislative framework,
- the state of the labour market,
- public expectations of employers,

- government policy,
- trade union power,
- European social policy, and
- sector and organizational culture.

Staff in the health service were, before the recent reforms, employed in the main by District Health Authorities. Those staff held contracts of employment based on nationally negotiated Whitley Council terms and conditions or on rates recommended by the review bodies. As a public service, with delegated budgets, employment in the health sector was reasonably secure. This scene has altered significantly. Staff in the health service are now typically employed by NHS Trusts, perhaps on Whitley terms which have been inherited but increasingly on local terms. Staff are also now inextricably linked to an output and so cannot be separated from its price. As Trusts have no guarantee that the services they provide will be purchased, so staff have become a semi-variable rather than a fixed cost; or at least the fragility of employment in Trusts has been highlighted. More positively, in a service where purchasers have choices, staff with their skills and reputations become part of any Trust's unique competitive advantage. Without the right number of staff with the skills needed a Trust's capacity to attract work or to deliver quality care is impaired.

The human resources agenda

Given the context described above, managers are faced (as suggested) with a new agenda for staff management which extends beyond selection interviewing, induction, appraisal and other such traditional personnel activities. This new agenda includes:

- employee resourcing,
- human resource planning,
- organization structure,
- labour utilization,
- reward,
- employee relations, and
- performance.

Employee resourcing

Sustaining a large service organization which relies on a wide range of specialist skills means ensuring the supply of, recruiting, training and retaining the right numbers of staff of the disciplines required. Managers, therefore, must address sources of labour and the recruitment, selection and induction of that labour. The entry, maintenance and exit of staff from services are clearly real management concerns which will be explored.

Human resource planning

An essential part of service business planning is the staff element. Information regarding the current stock of human resources is a necessary starting point. From employment records managers can examine variables such as numbers of staff in different categories, turnover, coming retirements, absence, wage costs and so on. When this information is related to the future service demands, the workforce level and configuration can be planned and controlled to best effect.

Organization structure

Service managers have to design employees' working structures and relationships taking into account needs for management control and clinical autonomy. The health service is made up of many professions each with their own identity, codes of practice and cultural traditions. These factors make the leadership role of health service managers difficult but essential.

Labour utilization

Staff costs account for such a high proportion of total costs that the best return on the money invested in staff is essential in a competitive market. Health service managers must design work processes to ensure labour is best utilized to maintain or increase productivity.

Reward

The health service reforms have given managers a new set of problems and challenges in devolving decision-making about pay, terms and conditions. What this means is that the reward for the job done lies in the hands of service managers alongside responsibility for the costs.

Employee relations

The individual and collective relationship between staff and their employer, as represented by managers, is a critical part of the success of any service. These relationships operate at different levels (whether they be individual or with the group) and they operate at different levels of formality, including contact with trade unions. Managers need to maintain a healthy relationship with and between their staff.

Performance

Performance management, or getting the best from staff, almost defines the management task. This goes beyond setting objectives or appraisal and requires a holistic approach including considering what motivates the health service worker.

Empowerment of managers

Much of the essential thinking about the above areas of policy and practice presently takes place inside personnel departments. This seems strange if not uncomfortable. A clear fact that faces managers is that they manage, and this includes management of their personnel. Spencer (1967) stated

'The Minister of Health is quoted as saying he is not sure that the introduction of personnel officers is the right approach to good personnel management in hospitals, and asking whether there may not be risks in appearing to take responsibility for staff management out of the hands of managers and supervisors on the spot. If staff relations are not as good as they might be, might the remedy not be to provide better opportunities for departmental heads and supervisors to be trained in the techniques of personnel management?'

Recent writing on human resource management (HRM) emphasizes the key role of managers, indeed Guest (1991) said 'HRM is too important to be left to personnel managers'. Hence the original idea for this book. There may be doubt whether first-line managers, to whom the book is addressed, are likely to have the freedoms envisaged by the suggested Activities and possibly some first-line managers will not be motivated to read a book with such a strong slant to personnel. However, the health service described earlier in this chapter demands that managers take control of the personnel agenda. The people involved and the environment that the new structures create will ensure enthusiastic agenda ownership.

So how does the health service reach a position where managers allow others, finance advisors, planners, personnel officers etc., to do some of their job for them. The question is retrospective as general management is foreign to the health service, the NHS dominant culture is one of professionalism, specialization and demarcation.

Many health service managers, who may have come from one of the professions themselves, feel they owe their allegiance to that profession. Specific management training for health service managers is fairly new and as yet not sufficiently recognized or widely taken up. Conversely, for example, accountancy and personnel management are established professions with supporting institutes and qualifications. Health service managers in previous roles have been all too ready to accept the direct intervention and assistance of these supporting management professions. Recent trends towards empowerment and decentralization are changing the situation.

Management audit

The simple audit tool given below is designed to help managers self-assess whether they manage staff themselves or to what extent they allow this to be done for them by specialist personnel officers. It selects an activity in which all managers are involved, that is recruitment. The results will probably show a balance of responses in either column. Managers should take a view about how much they are allowing to be done for them against what they should undertake themselves.

Activity

Consider the role of line managers in recruitment in your service.

Tick below the column that applies in each instance.

Task completed by:	Line Manager	Personnel Officer
(1) Reviewing the vacancy	☐	☐
(2) Writing job advertisements	☐	☐
(3) Calling candidates for interview	☐	☐
(4) Making and obtaining acceptance of offer	☐	☐
(5) Sending for references and arranging medical screening	☐	☐
(6) Informing unsuccessful candidates	☐	☐
(7) Contract preparation/ signing, collecting P45 and bank details etc.	☐	☐
(8) Providing instructions to payroll services for salary	☐	☐
(9) Induction management	☐	☐

If the ticks are all in one column it is not necessarily right, nor indeed wrong. For example, it may be appropriate to have a personnel officer relieve managers of the more time consuming aspects of a staffing process, e.g. calling candidates for interview. Indeed, much of the process described above could be left to a personnel officer if certain key points are held by management; these are deciding on the job to be done, making the appointment decision and arranging appropriate induction. If, however, the ticks in the personnel column indicate a wider abdication of the role then rethinking may be appropriate. Conversely, finding a list of line manager ticks may indicate agenda ownership or inappropriate delegation.

Of course, the examples given in the checklist above may seem in themselves somewhat mundane. If the table included deciding on job content or selecting the successful candidate the test may yield different results.

Summary

The health service is a unique service provided by a unique set of organizations. Recent changes to both the structure and culture of the provision of health services impact directly on its managers. In parallel, personnel management has changed its focus in organizations. As health services now operate in a competitive environment and rely on skilled staff resources, which absorb a significant majority of the money available, personnel management becomes a key issue. Managers of health services need to address the new health environment as general managers in a real sense and have a clear view of their employed human resources.

This book looks at personnel management:

- as a practical set of business tools,
- as an issue for general managers rather than specialists,
- in a health context, and
- in the light of employment and health reforms.

References

Guest, D.E. (1991) Personnel Management: the end of orthodoxy. *British Journal of Industrial Relations*, 29, **2**, 149–76.

Johnson, G. & Scholes, K. (1988) *Exploring Corporate Strategy*. Prentice Hall.

Likert, R. (1967), *The Human Organisation: Its Management and Value*. McGraw Hill Book Company, New York.

Spencer, J.A. (1967) *Management in Hospitals*. Faber and Faber, London.

Chapter 2:
EMPLOYEE RESOURCING

Introduction

One of the most visible or obvious personnel management roles conducted by managers is the 'hiring and firing' of staff. This is also the part of the management task which creates a regular link between managers and personnel department specialists in providing some form of support. This chapter will take the whole cycle of a resignation from post, recruiting a replacement by making an appointment and then following up that appointment, to the new employee leaving the organization. The cycle described forms the foundation for many of the policies, procedures and actions covered in the rest of the book.

Learning outcomes

- To understand why people leave an organization, the methods and importance of discovering their reasons for leaving.

- To appreciate the stages involved in the recruitment and selection process, the investment that process represents and the need to make a good decision.

- To understand the process of appointment and induction, once someone is found who is to join the organization.

- To see the critical place of providing for equality of opportunity at every stage of the employment process.

- To understand the legal and procedural context that surrounds people leaving employment either through choice or compulsion.

Staff leaving voluntarily

Exit interviews

When employees wish to leave an organization they are required to give notice, normally in writing, stating that they are ending the employment relationship. This period of notice is specified in each employee's contract of employment and in statute and will often coincide with the pay period, i.e. a week or a month. Some more senior appointments (or with longer service) demand longer periods of notice from the employee.

Existing staff may decide to leave their employment by resignation for a variety of reasons:

- maternity,
- retirement,
- returning to education,
- no longer needing or wanting to work,
- relocation of family, or
- having another job to go to.

Less frequently staff may leave not because of some positive factor but because they are dissatisfied with some aspect of their existing employment:

- lack of prospects,
- unsatisfactory environment,
- relationships with colleagues, or
- insufficient variety of work.

A certain number of leavers from a work population is natural, and indeed beneficial, and cannot be avoided for the reasons given in the first list above. However, managers should be concerned if staff leave because of negative reasons within the workplace. An exit interview or questionnaire can be used while the employee is in the notice period in order to establish the reason for leaving. If any negative factors do exist a constructive discussion with the leaver can help the manager in taking corrective action before any new appointment arrives.

So one benefit of conducting an exit interview is to establish the background reasons for leaving.

Other benefits flowing from interviewing a leaver will include the chance both to update or transfer knowledge about the post before the existing expertise departs and to find out what skills the leaver had which meant they could successfully do the job. It is also most important to say 'thank you' to the employee, leaving a good image of the organization in the employee's mind. Such interviews are best conducted informally, soon after the resignation is made, and should include an assurance that whatever is said will not affect the employee's work record or future references.

This interview is best conducted by the immediate line manager. Personnel specialists may then undertake a statistical analysis of all leavers and feed that data back to managers. Departmental personnel specialists may maintain that they should undertake exit interviews for all staff or directly receive the results of exit questionnaires. The rationale for this is that the employee may be leaving because of the manager which would not be discovered in a manager-led interview. However, the incidence of negative reasons for leaving relating to management behaviour is so small it does not tip the balance in favour of personnel specialist-led exit interviews.

Resignation checklist

When staff tender their resignation do you:

Conduct an exit interview ☐

Provide an exit questionnaire ☐

Refer to Personnel for processing ☐

What happens, if anything, to the information from exit interviews?

Leaver administration

The employee who is leaving, given the notice period, will have provided or will be waiting to hear when their last day on duty is to be. If the employee still has outstanding annual leave entitlement this either can be taken prior to the contract end date, so bringing forward the last day on duty, or can be paid.

If the employee was making payments into the NHS pension

scheme repayment of contributions or retention of benefits may be required. The employee will also need to be provided with a form to let any future employer know the tax position (P45).

Some employing organizations have a policy of positively recognizing long service by making an award or presentation to the member of staff which may happen at the same time as some form of social function. The manager, informed by the organization's policy and practice, should decide how to mark staff departures.

Recruitment and selection

The process of finding a replacement for any leaver is not short. As soon as a notice of resignation is given the line managers should consider the need, or not, for a replacement. Should a replacement be required a broad view of the typical replacement timescales might be:

Stage	Typical timescale
Conduct exit interview	1
Review the post	5
Prepare job description	1
Prepare personnel specification	1
Prepare and place advertisement	8
Closing date	7
Shortlising for interview	4
Interview notification	7
Pre-employment checks	7
Offer of employment	2
Notice period potentially required	30
Total process	**73 days**

While three months may seem a long time, each time gap is in itself reasonable and justifiable. A weekly publication, with press deadlines, may mean eight days before the job advertisement appears (some publications are monthly). Candidates need at least a week to respond to an advertisement by requesting, completing and returning an application form; they also need a week's notice of their interview to be able to attend. Health service pre-employment screening can be detailed and may often take more than a week. Successful candidates already in employment will have themselves to give notice. While posts can be filled within the time periods identified some can take much longer; for example, if the post requires re-grading, or advertisement in a specialist journal is sought, or the candidate has to give longer notice than indicated here.

What this timetable highlights is that recruitment is a long and expensive process. It is important that the process is efficient and cost effective. Unnecessary delay between the notice of resignation and thinking about a replacement will delay the eventual appointment. At the same time line managers can challenge the process to produce a quicker, more flexible response from personnel specialists.

Vacancy scrutiny

There is also the possibility that the post is no longer required at all, or that the funds released could be spent on completely new staffing solutions.

The first task of the manager, before authorising any further work on recruitment, is to establish that replacement is really required and there is funding to support it. A vacancy presents the manager with choices about the vacant post and other posts around it. As the organization's needs change so vacancies can be used to re-organize the way work is done to meet those changing needs. The post may have changed since it was last filled in its purpose, position, location or responsibilities. The options set out below should be considered.

Vacancy scrutiny checklist

Re-allocation of the work to others in the organization ☐

Restructuring to absorb the duties so losing the post ☐

Transfer of an employee from elsewhere whose present post is at risk ☐

Changing the duties ☐

Recruitment to the post as it stands ☐

Chapter 3 on Human Resource Planning will introduce methodologies by which managers can make informed decisions about vacant posts.

Case study – vacancy scrutiny

A team of three contract managers and three information assistants have a secretary who has submitted her resignation. The roles of all the organization's employees had changed in the previous six months with the introduction of a computer network and extensive staff training on word processing and software packages. Many staff were now performing their own secretarial duties, e.g. typing, electronic mail and diaries. The team has to decide whether or not to replace the departing member of staff and if so how to define any new role.

If the post is not replaced remaining duties may be ignored or re-allocated to existing staff with a possible loss of efficiency. To replace with another secretary risks inefficient use of the resource represented by the post and of the skills of the secretary, so leading to job dissatisfaction.

Looking back at the checklist above, consider how you would go about helping the team to decide what they should do about the approaching departure of their existing secretary.

Job description and personnel specification

The scrutiny of the post will give a clearer idea of what the organization requires which will enable the job to be 'described'. Job descriptions carry a set of information which, while still a *précis* of the complexity of any role, can be helpful to the manager and prospective candidates. Job descriptions should include the items shown below.

Job description checklist

Post title ☐

Main purpose of the job ☐

Department ☐

Location ☐

Grade ☐

Responsibility for staff	☐
Responsibility for budget	☐
Authority	☐
Scope of accountability	☐
Duties or objectives	☐

As well as serving as a basis for the personnel specification to assist recruitment and training needs analysis, job descriptions are also helpful in:

- reviewing performance,
- identifying training needs,
- grading posts,
- reviewing organizational structures, and
- demonstrating previous experience.

Job descriptions become unhelpful if they are task orientated and so become limiting for individuals or organizations in their literal interpretation.

'Personnel specifications' simply convert the identified job requirements in the job description into individual attributes so that a candidate can be selected who fits the job requirements. Previous experience, qualifications, personal characteristics and so on will read across from the job description. Other factors which may influence the personnel specification include the fit of an individual into the existing team and organizational values. The criteria must, however, be strictly relevant to the job to avoid any equal opportunities difficulties. Clearly, personal features must not include age, gender, race, marital status or physical requirements (above the minimum requirements).

Two forms of personnel specification commonly used are the Seven Point Plan produced by Alec Rodger of the National Institute of Industrial Psychology and John Munro Fraser's Five-fold Grading System.

The Seven Point Plan

1. Physical make-up or requirements.
2. Attainments.

3. General intelligence.
4. Special aptitudes.
5. Interests.
6. Disposition.
7. Circumstances.

Five-fold Grading System

1. Impact on others.
2. Acquired qualifications.
3. Innate abilities.
4. Motivation.
5. Adjustment.

It is important in using the above scales, or any other, to refine them by identifying:

● factors which are essential,
● factors which are desirable but not essential, and
● factors which would be contra-indications, i.e. they would take the individual out of further consideration.

Activity

Do all the staff who report to you have job descriptions and personnel specifications for the posts they hold?

If the answer is no, would it be prudent to prepare these documents while experienced staff are in-post?

Advertisement

Each geographical area has hundreds of employers, large and small, and a pool of labour which is unemployed, or seeking work other than the work they have. The employing health service organization has to make its own distinctive voice heard in this crowd so that it both finds potential candidates of the right calibre and attracts them sufficiently to apply. Aside from job-specific advertising the personnel specialist, if present, may maintain contact with the employment centre, careers officers and local schools; and also attend careers fairs to give the health service employer a presence and profile. The purpose of a job-specific advertisement is to attract applicants. Health organizations are usually large enough to have jobs every week and space can be held through an agency in the local paper so the public know the day the advertisement will appear containing that week's jobs.

If the applicant base available is likely to be large, or at least sufficient, the advertisement might seek to discourage unsuitable applicants by setting out some of the screening criteria that will be used. Advertisement text is expensive so it should be written to contain factual and relevant information. The style is as important as the content in getting and keeping the right candidates' attention; this may include position on the page. Advertisements should not include anything which directly or indirectly discriminates on grounds of gender, marital status, race, ethnic origin, trade union membership or disability, unless such content is clearly related to an essential job requirement which is recognized as being excluded from the relevant Acts.

Places for advertisements to be seen, once created, might include:

- national and local newspapers,
- professional journals,
- employment centres,
- universities or colleges,
- recruitment agencies,
- careers services,
- public noticeboards, and
- internal vacancy bulletins.

Information should be available on the cost and previous success rates for each of these media, and in some cases their readership, client base or coverage. Advertising should, at the same time, be consistent with the health service organization's corporate image and values.

Applications

The advertisement wording should make it clear to such readers who decide they are interested and suitable how they are to respond. It could ask that they:

- send a *curriculum vitae,*
- telephone for an application form,
- telephone for an informal conversation, or
- arrange to visit.

The most common and straightforward method used is to ask candidates to telephone for an application form to complete and return before a pre-determined closing date. Such forms allow the manager to collect standard and consistent information about each candidate in a single format for easy reference and comparison. They speed sorting and shortlisting against set criteria and make a good starting point for any future personnel record. As well as sending the applicant a blank application form to complete and return the opportunity may be taken to provide further and better particulars about the job. These may include:

- the job description,
- the personnel specification,
- a profile of the department or organization, and
- an organizational structure chart.

Shortlisting

Many applications for posts are from hopeful but unsuitable candidates who need to be screened out before the real process of selection begins. This process of thinning out is often called 'shortlisting'. The criteria used to shortlist should be applied equally to all the applicants. It is common for managers to shortlist application forms on the basis of the amount written, handwriting, grammar or neatness. However, such factors should only be used if a test of literacy or presentation is a genuine requirement of the job. As far as possible the application form should seek factual data which can be checked i.e. qualifications, previous experience, duties of current posts and so on. Asking open questions and expecting candidates to fill page space is inviting them to use their imagination and to write things that sound impressive but have little shortlisting value. At the other extreme, however, simple, factual responses are simply not enough to base shortlisting decisions on.

Selection

Having shortlisted a set of candidates who, on a crude analysis of essential attributes, could fill the vacant job finer judgments must be made. In selection the manager needs to be able to predict which is likely to be the most successful candidate in the job and select that one. Some pseudo-scientific methods of predicting job success such as astrology or graphology amount in reality to little more than complete chance prediction. The bad news is that no available predictive technique provides a perfect job performance prediction. That is, no available selection technique produces an absolute correlation between the prediction of future job success made at the time of selection and subsequent reality. Techniques for selection include:

- assessment centres,
- team problem solving exercises,
- work sample tests e.g. an in-tray exercise,
- ability tests e.g. numerical reasoning,
- comprehension e.g. understanding mechanical ideas,
- aptitude tests e.g. capacity to acquire a particular skill,
- attainment tests e.g. acquired mathematical skills,
- personality tests e.g. introversion and extroversion,
- interviews (structured and unstructured), and
- references.

Most, if not all, managers choose to use an interview as their preferred means of selection. Even if the interviewer is trained and the interview well structured the predictive validity of selection interviewing is low. Forbes (1979) says:

> 'There is a tendency in this type of situation to wander from the main point of identifying variables that will indicate future success and the interview can degenerate into a "chat" session with the interviewer, if he is untrained, doing most of the "chatting".'

At this level the interview is likely to be no more successful than chance prediction.

Interviews

Despite the many critics of the interview (e.g. Eysenck 1953), it has always been preferred by managers selecting candidates for posts and so it is worth highlighting ways to make it more effective. There is a tendency for some managers to make their decisions in selection on the basis of personal subjective criteria which cannot be referred back to the criteria for the job.

The interview panel should be carefully selected so they know the job, can assess the candidate and make judgments without prejudice. Interviewing should always involve more than one assessor so the ideas and assumptions of one can be challenged by another after each interview. Also, one can focus on listening to the answers while another asks questions. For medical appointments there is little room for local discretion in selection as appointment committee membership is laid down. Consultant appointments in England and Wales, for example, are governed by the provisions of the NHS (Appointment of Consultant) Regulations 1982 and appointment panels have to consist of:

- lay chairman,
- Royal College representative,
- university representative,
- regional adviser,
- medical director,
- speciality representative,
- chief executive, and
- lay member.

The interview should be structured so each candidate experiences, as far as possible, a similar test and the interviewers have a like basis for comparison. To achieve this the interviewers should meet and prepare the interviews before they take place to ensure that they each know their specific role and topic area.

A means of assessment or recording of each candidate's replies is necessary so that the product of each interview is objective rather than based on memory.

The questions should be about facts rather than interpretation, past performance rather than hypothetical behaviour, and specific rather than general. Questions should not allow 'yes' or 'no' answers and should not be leading or suggestive of the answer sought.

The recording of interview findings is important to:

- aid recall,
- allow objective assessment,
- ensure the agreed criteria are covered,
- make comparisons,
- give feedback,
- justify decisions later, and
- use for evaluation purposes.

By extending the personnel specification the manager can

decide the selection methods which are necessary to distinguish between the candidates. For example, if an acquired qualification is essential it can be identified by looking at the application form, asking for sight of a certificate or testing directly for the knowledge required.

The appointment decision

Following on from the assessment of candidates and predictions of how they would perform in the job a selection decision has to be made. At the same time as the panel makes its selection decision, so the candidates will be making judgments on the basis of what they have seen. Each selection technique used should have produced results which have been recorded in a standardized way for each candidate. Each candidate should be considered in turn in an objective way by the decision-makers to reach a view on relative results. The decisions regarding each should be recorded giving reasons for acceptance or rejection; this is for possible feedback to the candidates on their performance.

In the health service reaching the stage of selecting the most suitable candidate for the job is not the end of the process. Careful pre-employment screening has to precede any employment offer. This may include:

- taking up employment references,
- medical (occupational health) screening,
- the screening of criminal records for staff working with children,
- taking up general practitioner references,
- professional registration checks, and
- checking work permits.

Offer of employment

The basis of the employment relationship between employer and employee is the individual contract of employment. The employment contract is not just the paper documentation; a statutory requirement exists that all employees receive or have sight of a principal statement describing important elements of the contract, but this does not cover its whole scope. The contract is formed as an agreement between the employer and employee on the basis of an offer and acceptance. When a telephone call is made or an offer letter written to the favoured candidate a clear intention exists to enter an agreement which is to be legally binding. If accepted the offer in its details becomes part of the legal contract. Managers making employment offers should be well prepared, understand what they are offering and be clear on the limits on their flexibility to reach agreement. Such information may include:

- salary,
- main terms and conditions e.g. hours,
- duties,
- start date,
- where to report on the first day,
- sickness and holiday procedures, and
- relocation assistance.

Managers should ensure, where it is possible, that their future actions are not restricted by inflexible contract terms.

If the preferred candidate accepts the offer this should be followed by:

- a formal letter of appointment,
- the principal statement of terms, and
- a staff handbook, if appropriate.

The manager will need to obtain details from the future employee including bank account details, tax information (P45 or P46), birth certificate and national insurance number.

The manager, on behalf of the employer, becomes responsible for meeting certain implicit or common law duties in employing the successful candidate. For example, the manager should take reasonable care to protect the health of the employee at work. The employer may become liable vicariously for any faults or misdeeds on the part of the manager in relation to the employee in their work. The employee must be paid and provided with the work necessary to maintain specialist skills. The employee for their part must, on entering into the contract, give faithful service and should not act to substantially harm the employer; and so must not work for a competitor or compete directly. The contract of employment is personal and so the employee must attend work in person and cannot send a substitute.

Induction

Managers should ensure a new employee receives a planned induction within the workplace, starting on the first day. Very obvious needs exist from the employee's point of view; to know where they are to work, who they will be working with, where the toilets are, any safety rules and what happens in case of a fire. But such basic survival information is really not in itself adequate to ensure the employee's success. Induction should:

- welcome the new employee and help them identify with their new place of work,
- engender a feeling of commitment and responsibility,
- familiarize the employee with the organization, its purpose, aims and methods of working,
- provide support in settling into the job and meeting its demands, and
- indicate the standard of performance required.

More specifically, the manager should:

- arrange for someone to act as the new employee's 'friend' or 'mentor' in their first months,
- brief existing staff on the new recruit's arrival,
- ensure working space and equipment is available, and
- give a clear start time and location to the recruit for them to be met and welcomed.

The health professions through preceptorship, mentoring or clinical supervision can manage induction in a structured way.

Key items to cover in the induction period would include those described below.

Induction checklist

Disciplinary rules ☐

Grievance procedure ☐

Confidentiality ☐

Protection of patients and their rights ☐

Fire procedure and precautions ☐

Security awareness ☐

Occupational health and safety ☐

Control of infection ☐

Lifting training ☐

Resuscitation skills ☐

Equal opportunities policies ☐

Activity

Think about your own induction to your job or the induction of your most recent joiner. How much of what is suggested above was provided to you or them?

Personal file

Employee's details are confidential and so should be kept in a single secure place with only appropriate controlled access. Once an employee has accepted a post the information set out below should exist to form the basis of their file.

Personal file checklist

Job advertisement ☐

Personnel specification ☐

Job description ☐

Application form ☐

Interview assessment record ☐

References ☐

Results of pre-employment screening ☐

Copy of any offer letter ☐

Principal statement of terms ☐

Induction checklist. ☐

Any further information or correspondence relating to the employee should also be stored in this one file. An obvious sign of the role confusion between line managers and personnel specialists arises in difficulty about where such information is to be kept and who owns it. Does having employee files locked away in a personnel department engender feelings of line management ownership?

Evaluating the process

The panel should meet following appointment to review the process to see if it could be improved or whether any lessons can be learnt. Of particular concern is whether the process provided the quality and quantity of information necessary to make the employment decision. If the interview assessment record shows whether the successful candidate exceeded all, most or some of the selection criteria, comparisons can now be made against actual performance in the job. Discrepancies between performance at selection and performance in post point to a need to think again about the criteria or selection methods used. Another sign of a poor selection process could be failure to keep new recruits through their induction i.e. more than three months.

The clear hope is that the candidate who is well informed about the position available and who performs well in selection tests goes on to become a happy motivated worker who performs well here too.

Equal opportunities

Recruitment may, at first, seem a strange place to talk about the inappropriateness of discrimination as the intention is to discriminate or discern between the attributes of individual candidates and select on the basis of that discrimination. It is the case that appropriate discrimination in a recruitment context is fair, for example on the basis of intelligence, experience or aptitudes, while other areas of discrimination are unfair or illegal. The areas of discrimination which are seen as unfair or illegal need to be considered from job advertisement through to pension payments.

Categories of discrimination

Under statute, managers should ensure no individual or group of individuals receives less favourable treatment or facilities on the grounds of gender, marital status, pregnancy, race, colour, nationality, ethnic origin or trade union membership. While outside of Northern Ireland specific statutory protection does not extend to religion, under the Race Relations Act 1976 it is also unlawful to discriminate against Sikhs and Jews (*Mandla* v. *Lee* (1983) and *Seide* v. *Gillette Industries* (1980)). Organizations may also have policies against discrimination on grounds of age, disability, religious belief, dependants or part-time worker status; although such is not necessarily illegal, unless involving indirect discrimination against the above mentioned groups. In Northern Ireland legislation against religious discrimination exists. Disabled persons do have the right not to be unfairly discriminated against supported by statute in the Disabled Persons (Employment) Acts 1944 and 1958 but they are not very effective in preventing discrimination and new legislation may be introduced in the future.

There are various forms of discrimination or victimization. Direct discrimination is not commonplace because it is action which is obvious in disadvantaging one group or individual over the other. More common forms of discrimination are indirect where a rule or requirement exists that cannot be justified and which a considerably smaller proportion of one race or gender can meet.

Below the level of policy, the behaviour of individuals can be discriminatory. Individuals or groups can be victimized, segregated, harassed or discouraged at work.

Employing organizations clearly have a responsibility to ensure that neither they nor their employees discriminate either in the narrow legal sense or in the wider ethical sense. Also, organizations should introduce arrangements in order to meet their obligations as employers.

Managers should ensure that they and all their staff are aware of:

- the areas of discrimination which are disallowed,
- when discrimination may occur, and
- the types of behaviour that would be considered discriminatory.

Managers should also ensure that any grievances or complaints of harassment are dealt with properly, fairly and as quickly as possible. Good social, economic and competitive reasons exist to eliminate discrimination, aside from the legal remedies that may be sought against such employers. In announcing a programme of action in relation to ethnic minorities and employment in December 1993, Mrs Virginia Bottomley, Secretary of State for Health, stated:

> '...taking action to promote equality in employment is not just a matter of moral justice or of fairness. It is good, sound common sense and it makes business sense too.'

Discrimination can occur at any time but particular attention should be paid to:

- advertising, recruitment and selection;
- engagement, pay, terms and conditions;
- access to training, promotion and career development;
- pregnancy and maternity leave; and
- dismissal or retirement.

Advertising, recruitment and selection

The wording in or presentation of job advertisements should not discourage or debar particular groups or individuals from making a response on grounds of their gender or race. The works department should not advertise for a 'handyman' but could call the same job a 'maintenance assistant'. Ward sister posts should be 'ward sister/charge nurse' to avoid any sexual connotation, or additional wording could be added saying that enquiries are welcomed from men and women.

Engagement, pay, terms and conditions

An offer of employment to a person of one gender or race on terms which are less favourable than those which had been or might be offered to others is clearly unlawful. Employers should provide the same pay and conditions to any employees doing the same or similar work of equal value.

Training, promotion and career development

Employing organizations should not discriminate unlawfully in granting access to training, allowing the pursuance of career opportunities or providing benefits for some individuals and not others based on illegal criteria. The treatment of part-time staff, who are more likely to be women, is of particular importance in this regard in order to avoid indirect discrimination.

Dismissal or retirement

Dismissing a woman because she is pregnant, likely to become pregnant, has changed her marital status or wishes to take maternity leave is unlawful. If continuing to employ a woman who is pregnant would endanger that woman or others then alternative work should be provided or suspension on full pay offered. Dismissing an employee who complained about harassment or discrimination would almost certainly be unlawful. Sex-based differences in retirement provision should be removed including differences in long service award entitlements.

Monitoring the diversity

Monitoring key areas such as the number of women or ethnic minorities who apply for posts, are shortlisted or are appointed, may be helpful in assessing whether managers are avoiding equal opportunities policies. It may also be helpful to monitor the progression of these groups and others within the organization. It serves to raise awareness of the issues and potential problem areas. The Opportunity 2000 targets and action plans suggest both monitoring and targets.

Such monitoring can be costly and time consuming. It can also cause apathy as the measurement is seen as action in and of itself. Monitoring can also be counterproductive in that awareness is raised about race, gender or disability so increasing the possibilities for discrimination. Organizations that attempt to record such data may find a proportion of their employees are unwilling to participate or provide such information about themselves for the reasons given above.

Simply having a written policy about equal opportunities is clearly not enough as it does not guarantee anything. Training, familiarization and persuasion are probably the most effective actions for managers to consider.

Case study – sex discrimination

A six month temporary position was advertised in a busy Medical Records Department. Following acceptance of an offer of employment the successful candidate told the Medical Records Manager she was 20 weeks pregnant and proposed in writing when she wished to take her maternity leave. The effect of combined annual leave and maternity leave would be that the successful candidate would only work the first half of the temporary six month period. Having established the candidate was aware of her pregnancy at interview but did not declare that fact to the selection panel the manager withdrew the offer of employment. The candidate made an application to Industrial Tribunal complaining the withdrawal of the job offer was due to pregnancy and so was direct sex discrimination. The manager maintained the temporary additional post was essential and required an occupant to attend for work during whole of the six month temporary period. Discuss the factors involved here and decide whether or not illegal discrimination has taken place.

The manager in this case study had a selection criterion of availability for work. That criterion could be applied to either gender and it could be shown that the criterion was justifiable. However, in similar cases the dismissal has been found to be unfair as the reason given was pregnancy.

Activity

Consider whether or not the mix of your staff represents the diversity of the population outside the organization in which you work.

Exceptions

In some special circumstances selection can involve discrimination in areas which would normally be considered illegal. For example, if a requirement exists for a postholder to be physically able to lift patients without the risk of a back injury then candidates' height/weight ratio may be taken into account even though height qualifications would be considered as indirect discrimination against women. Examples in this category are called genuine occupational qualifications and may exclude certain posts from the normal statutory requirements.

Ending the employment contract

The employment relationship can be terminated through the agreement (or mutual consent) of both parties, employer and employee, at any time. If only one party or other wishes to withdraw from the contract notice must be served on the other side. Minimum periods of notice are set out by statute but longer notice periods may be required by the employment contract. If the employee serves notice it is resignation: if the employer serves notice it is dismissal. If employees feel they have been forced into serving a notice of resignation it is considered to be 'constructive dismissal'. This occurs where the employer's actions have gravely breached the terms of the contract and the employee has no effective choice but to resign.

The employment contract can be ended without either party wishing to bring about the termination through 'a frustrating event'. That is, some event happens which is the fault of neither party but which makes the contract impossible to honour e.g. serious illness, imprisonment or statutory impediment (a driving ban). The employer can go bankrupt or go into liquidation which would have a similar effect but a redundancy claim would stand in that instance. To summarize the employment contract can be ended by:

- mutual consent,
- the employee's notice of resignation,
- the employer's notice of dismissal,
- 'frustration' by some event, or
- bankruptcy or liquidation of the employer.

Resignation by the employee is a fairly simple action. If the notice period given by the employee is too short, or no notice is given, then the employer can take legal action to seek damages. Employers rarely take such action because, even if such a claim were successful, the remedy would usually only be an award of the earnings payable in the notice period.

Dismissal is conversely a complex action which often

involves statutory protection providing rights to the employee. Depending on length of service, the employee has a real ability to seek redress if the employer's action is either wrongful or conducted in the wrong way. This can be either through an Industrial Tribunal claiming unfair dismissal or by pursuing action in the civil courts for wrongful dismissal in breach of the employment contract.

The employer can take dismissal action, with or without notice, because of the employee's misconduct, incapability or ill-health. If the employee's misconduct or incompetence is considered to be gross, then the employer need neither pay nor provide the notice required by statute or by the contract as it is the employee who is deemed to have repudiated the terms of that contract.

Dismissal can also come about through:

- redundancy,
- retirement,
- refusal to re-engage after industrial action which has broken the contract,
- refusal to renew a fixed-term contract,
- refusal to permit a return after pregnancy, or
- the employer acting to force a resignation.

In Chapter 7 on Employee Relations the procedures which regulate these dismissal actions in the employment relationship are examined.

Termination of employment

Employment can end without the employers having that as their intention or serving notice. In the case study below consider whether the employee was dismissed or whether the employment contract remained intact, and what led you to either conclusion.

Case study – termination of employment

A Community Care team had two management posts, Nurse Manager and Senior Nurse Manager, with one reporting to the other. Following a review and re-organization, two new and equal posts were proposed to replace the existing two management positions. The new positions divided the management and clinical aspects of the old roles so one was Manager, who need not be a nurse, and the other was Nursing and Quality Advisor, who did need a nursing background. Application forms for both posts were sent to the two existing postholders. The ex-Senior Nurse Manager applied for, was offered and accepted the post of Nursing and Quality Advisor on a protected salary. The Nursing Manager, who did not submit either application, was offered the remaining management position. The post was accepted under protest. The Nursing Manager subsequently claimed to have been dismissed because the new post removed any clinical responsibilities. The Trust maintained that the new posts were developments of the old ones and, as neither individual lost any income or status, no dismissal had taken place. Which is the correct position?

This case is interesting as the Nurse Manager could pursue a claim for unfair dismissal and, if on balance constructive dismissal took place and was unfair, would be entitled to a compensation award or reinstatement. It is unlikely, however, that any grave breach of the terms of the contract would be found, the changes being seen as simply variation of the contractual terms. The resignation would therefore be voluntary giving no rise to any rights other than to pay during the notice period.

Internal appeals

Health organizations tend to write into their procedures a facility for employees who find themselves given formal warnings or notice of dismissal to make an appeal against the managerial decision to impose such a sanction. A panel of managers senior to the manager with the authority to impose the original sanction hears the manager state why the decision was taken and the appellant states why the decision should be considered to be unfair or unreasonable. Internal appeals are important as they can correct faults in the originating disciplinary process. The appeal panel can:

● uphold the original decision,
● impose a different sanction which could be more or less severe,
● ask for a new disciplinary hearing to take place, or
● uphold the appeal in the employee's favour.

Industrial Tribunals

If the employer's action in dismissing the employee or the manner in which the dismissal was carried out is considered unfair by an Industrial Tribunal the remedies available to the employee include:

- re-instatement to the same position as held prior to the dismissal action,
- re-engagement on terms determined by the Tribunal, or
- compensation to cover lost benefits, wages and indeed lost future wages.

To make a claim of unfair dismissal employees must have met the service qualification, that is two years service.

In addition, the employee must have presented the claim to the Industrial Tribunal within three months of the effective date of the dismissal and must be no more than sixty-five years of age. Dismissal does not apply if the contract was a fixed-term contract which was not renewed and it contained an effective clause excluding an employee's rights to make any claim of dismissal on the basis of non-renewal.

The standards set by internal health service procedures which may lead to dismissal tend to ignore the statutory qualifications necessary to make a claim and so treat each individual equally. One of the tests Tribunals apply is whether or not employers, or their representatives, followed their own agreed procedures and whether such procedure was fair. Managers may find it inconvenient and unnecessary to treat an employee with one week's service with the same care as an employee with ten years' service but written internal procedures may not allow any distinction even though the employee could not make any claim.

Depending on the number of staff a manager has (and whether the manager is vested with authority to dismiss) experience of taking dismissal action may be limited. It is rare in the health service to give personnel specialists authority to dismiss unless they are acting as line managers within their own department, such authority tends to rest with a senior line manager who is bound to take the advice of a specialist and to follow a laid down procedure.

Each case really does need careful consideration on its own merits. The manager should, however, at all times act reasonably and fairly. A temptation exists to act too quickly without all the facts and this temptation must be resisted.

If managers feel they cannot continue to have an employee at work then suspension may be appropriate to allow an investigation and a return to duty or to a formal hearing.

If managers are to be involved in recruitment or dismissal, without the direct involvement of a personnel specialist, they should have received some training. The minimum requirement of the training would be to understand the basic statutory demands which, if not followed, would result in legal action against the employer.

Recommended further reading

Guidance is given by the Advisory, Conciliation and Arbitration Service in *Discipline at Work, The ACAS Advisory Handbook* (1987), and *Croner's Guide to Managing Fair Dismissal* (1993), Croner Publications Limited, is also helpful.

References

Forbes, R. (1979) Improving the Reliability of the Selection Interview. *Personnel Management* July 1979, 36–9.

Eysenck, H.J. (1953) *Uses and Abuses of Psychology.* Penguin, Harmondsworth.

Bottomley, V., Secretary of State for Health (1993) *Ethnic minority staff in the NHS: a programme of action.* NHS Management Executive, Department of Health.

Further information

Equal Opportunities Commission
Overseas House
Quay Street
Manchester
M3 3HN   Tel. 0161-833 9244

Commission for Racial Equality
Elliot House
Allington Street
London
SW1E 5EH   Tel. 0171-828 7022

Chapter 3:
HUMAN RESOURCE PLANNING

Introduction

A rationale for planning

Planning is clearly a management function. As the proverb goes: 'If we don't change the direction in which we are going, we might finish up where we are headed'. Health service organizations undertake planning at various levels, whether it be strategic, business or operational planning. Trusts must look for a realistic vision of their future, responding to external influences, changing markets and government policy. People, as a factor, must be part of those plans both to inform the possible and predict the consequences. Health organizations are staff-reliant and staff-intensive; any management plan has an impact on employment. Any Trust, or Trust sub-unit, needs to have plans which:

- ensure best utilization of existing resources,
- predict future resource requirements,
- project the capability of existing resources,
- avoid any over or under supply, and
- enable today's decisions to be based on tomorrow.

Mathis and Jackson (1988) state:

'In planning for human resources, an organisation must consider the allocation of people to jobs over long periods – not just for the next month or even the next year.'

Managers are often expected to write about people and employment in their business, speciality or directorate annual business plans. These workforce sections seldom in practice extend beyond a couple of paragraphs describing the current aggregate of staff employed with a repetition of one or two staff policies on, say, skill-mix. A greater level of sophistication amongst service managers in human resource planning is required to help those services achieve greater success and avoid the unnecessary human and financial costs resulting from unplanned or ill-considered change.

Learning outcomes

- To appreciate the information available to managers about the workforce that can be used for planning purposes, the means of managing and the importance of protecting that data.

- To understand in context the methodologies that can be developed to model data using assumptions about the future.

- To see the need for the workforce to be planned and managed against workload in a flexible and pro-active way.

- To see workforce data as an indicator of performance or as a means of organizational diagnosis.

What is planning?

Planning is concerned with:

- making predictions about the anticipated future,
- making decisions about the ideal future sought, and
- the interventions required to achieve what is desired.

In staff terms planning is concerned with the future work to be done, the methods of work and the staff needed, expressed as future demand for staff. Secondly, staff planning is concerned with ensuring an adequate supply of the skills required; or alternatively, if the supply is not sufficient, with changing the way work is planned to be done. Much of the planning so described is numerical and some is factual, but given the imponderables surrounding the future much planning is based on 'best guesses'.

Given a reasonable view of the future as it is predicted (and desired) decisions can be made to influence the future in line with the plan. Management is then less concerned with solving today's problems but rather with controlling the future.

This chapter aims to assist managers in developing simple manpower plans for their team, department or directorate, and then in making judgments on these for their annual business plans. It aims to assist managers in considering the consequences of plans or of planning and to use information available to them in decision-making.

Information

The importance of integration

All planning relies on a good supply of information about the business and its environment. Workforce information is a valuable resource which should be provided to and used by all levels of management. Like any resource, information needs to be managed. Workforce information needs to be managed as an organizational resource, for the benefit of the corporate whole, to directly improve management decision-making. It should be managed in a way consistent with the way the organization is managed by integrating manpower information into wider organizational planning. An integrated approach will ensure all the organization's resources are better utilized.

Good information is at the heart of any planning and human resource planning is no exception. Information can be used to inform, diagnose problems, assess performance, make judgments and to plan the future.

Internal and external data

A list of possible information requirements for human resource planning might be current and historical data about:

- staff numbers and whole-time equivalents,
- staff grades,
- locations,
- length of service,
- staff ages,
- staff gender,
- absenteeism,
- staff turnover,
- skills and qualifications held,
- workload,
- staff costs (basic and additional),
- sources of recruits,
- destinations of leavers, and
- patterns of work.

Other useful external information to supplement the above might include:

- unemployment statistics,
- local competition for labour,
- patterns of employment in the area,
- out-turn by local education providers,
- population movements, and
- impact of government reports.

Computers

The personnel department may utilize a computer to hold the above information to which line managers should also have access. Once information needs have been established for planning purposes the manager needs to consider:

- what systems will deliver that information,
- how reliability can be ensured, and
- how information is to be collected, stored, extracted and manipulated.

Computers store, sort, analyse and give fast, flexible access to information. Computerized personnel information systems may undertake basic administrative personnel tasks as well as giving planning capability. In looking for a suitable system, managers are often met in today's market with a bewildering range of alternatives and prices. Cost is a major concern when investing in a system, the three obvious costs being hardware, software and maintenance. There are other less obvious costs such as training, set-up, space and consumables, e.g. paper and disks. Another consideration must be the cost, or loss, of buying a system inappropriate to its purpose, which a clear specification of purpose will avoid.

It is helpful to categorize the essential attributes sought from a potential system which would meet the needs identified, and to look at the systems, within set costs, that meet the specifications. Such specifications may include:

- data capacity,
- speed of processing,
- compatibility with other systems,
- access,

- security, and
- functions.

The package to drive the hardware can be purchased as an 'off the shelf' standard personnel package or it can be written to suit the particular needs identified in the specification. The programme package will come with user instructions or an operating manual. Some organizations will install a demonstration version of a package on existing hardware for a trial period to inform the purchasing decision.

Data protection

The Data Protection Act 1984 is not concerned with manual employee records. Once those records are computerized by managers, even only for their own staff, then compliance with the Act is necessary. Personal data about employees should be held for a specified and declared purpose; the data should be accurate, kept up to date and kept only as long as is relevant to the stated purpose; and it should only be disclosed in a manner compatible with the purpose. In addition to those matters concerning the data itself the employees named, or those identifiable against any stored data item, should have access to it at reasonable intervals without undue delay and have the right to have such information corrected or erased if it is inaccurate.

Managers need to register their data, either through their Trust or directly with the Data Protection Registrar. Managers should also inform their employees if personal data is to be held on computer and supply a copy of that information, including an explanation of any data held in a coded form.

The only exception to these disclosure rules which is relevant to planning is data which describes the intentions of management. Such intentions may include computer-held plans concerning promotion, redundancy, retirement or redeployment.

Manual or paper-based records are not covered by this Act and no employee right of access exists.

Planning

Stocks and flows

One of the simplest workforce plans projects a service demand for staff into the future. Managers are often asked to predict their demand for care professionals in five years time to inform decisions about commissioning professional education from external providers and to help financial planning. The model described in Table 3.1 may assist in this task. The staff could be paediatric nurses, operating department practitioners, or any other health professional.

Table 3.1   Demand forecasting table

Year	One	Two	Three	Four	Five
Stock	50	50	48	52	58
Intake	10	10	12	16	20
Losses	10	12	8	10	12
Balance	50	48	52	58	66
Requirements	50	55	60	65	70
Additional demand	—	**7**	**8**	**7**	**4**

Each row of figures in Table 3.1 is explained below.

Stock

The current number of staff employed, usually expressed as whole time equivalents or numbers of heads, is needed to start. The figures in years two on to five are estimated within the table (taking forward the balance figure) but the first figure in year one has to be factual, in the case above the stock of current staff is 50.

Intake

In previous years demand will have been forecast and the numbers in training locally will reflect the demand predictions made in the past. The numbers in the intake row reflect the predicted out-turn from the appropriate education provider of the type of staff required or the part of that out-turn designated to the service in question. In the example given demand was increased last year so there is increasing out-turn from the programme in year three and in the subsequent two years.

Losses

Historical turnover rates, that is the numbers of leavers as a percentage of the staff in post, alongside a list of the ages of existing staff will enable a prediction of future leaver numbers shown as losses across the year columns.

Balance

By starting from 'stock' and adding the recruits and subtracting the leavers a balance is obtained which without further intervention will be the stock in future years. This figure is shown as the balance and is lifted up into the next year's stock to begin the calculation again.

Requirements

By examining workload predictions, service changes and possible future purchasing intentions regarding a service, it is possible to predict the staffing level actually required to deliver the work in the future. In the example above a steady growth in the staff numbers required is predicted. Staff requirements are examined in greater detail below (see Table 3.2, Hospital clinic staff requirements).

Additional demand

The last row is the difference between the 'balance' which is likely to be the stock available and that predicted as really required. Table 3.1 shows a shortfall in supply of skilled staff over the planning period. The manager can make a judgment that the additional numbers over and above those available from the local education provider might be recruited from a wider geography or from the existing unemployed pool of those skills seeking work locally. Alternatively, plans for the service expansion may have to be delayed until numbers in training can be expanded or work patterns changed to reduce reliance on the skill in short supply. The consequent thinking cannot take place without the initial analysis. Computer spreadsheets allow such tables to be changed quickly when new information or variables are added.

Staff requirements

Table 3.1 suggested that managers might need to examine workload predictions to forecast staffing levels required in future years. Investigation into the organization and its culture,

working practices and structure will show how labour is organized. Further examination of productivity, contract targets,
business plans, income and expenditure accounts will show
what the organization might be achieving or be expected to
achieve. Balancing these information components together and
creating forecasts based on predicted demand will indicate the
future shape of the organization. In the example given in Table
3.2 it is predicted that the work load will reduce because of a
purchaser intention to localize work from the acute hospital
dermatology centre into local health clinics operated by general
practitioners. In addition to a loss of referrals as the local clinics
begin operating, the hospital clinic is concurrently expected to
increase productivity, so releasing savings on its remaining
work. The hospital strategy is, in the example, to see its prices
fall and to exaggerate the costs gap between its services and the
community clinics which, although local, are more expensive.

Table 3.2   Hospital clinic staff requirements

Year	One	Two	Three	Four
Patient numbers	10 000	9 000	8 000	7 000
Staff requirements based on patient numbers	20	18(2)	16(4)	14(6)
Staff saving from planned productivity increase	—	1	1(2)	1(3)
Total staff	20	17(3)	14(6)	11(9)

Figures in brackets ( ) indicate the cumulative totals of staff savings.
Each row of figures in Table 3.2 is explained below.

Patient numbers
> The centre manager believes that over the four year planning
> period 3 000 patients will be lost to community clinics at a
> steady rate of loss and this is shown in the first row.

Staff requirements based on patient numbers
> Given that 20 staff were required to run 10 000 patients the ratio
> can be applied down the line giving a reduction of two each

year, with a cumulative total of six staff lost. In larger examples the staff numbers required may have a 'step' rather than a 'straight-line' relationship to workload. For example, if activity falls enough to close a bed or a ward those are steps down which release staff unevenly.

Staff saving from planned productivity increase

The internal hospital efficiency savings programme and the need to be price competitive demand increased productivity in respect of the remaining workload by reducing staff by one each year, a cumulative total of three over the planning period.

Total staff reductions

Taking into account the fall in workload and the staff savings expected the new total stock can be forecast. It is from this type of calculation that the figure which goes into the demand forecasting table (Table 3.1) in the 'requirements' row is reached. In the first example staff were in under-supply by the training provider affecting expansion plans on the timescale envisaged. In the last example the level of leavers that might be predicted to occur naturally may not be enough for the staff reductions required.

Changing patterns

Flexibility

The market for public health care is no longer in a steady state. Trusts are faced with fluctuating needs or demands and have to change the levels and patterns of service provision. Traditional health service employment patterns, involving large numbers of permanent full-time jobs with high levels of contractual protection against organizational change make such market driven changes painful. New employment practices are being introduced which better match the health service of the annual contract for care provision. As purchasers move more and more of a Trust's funding into non-recurring or variable contracts, so the Trust carrying an increased risk must react by changing its cost base. Such initiatives may include greater use being made of:

- the self-employed,
- bank workers ('as and when required' contracts),

- agency staff,
- short-term/temporary contracts, and
- part-time contracts.

Increasingly the pattern of set working hours and permanently employed labour can be seen as an inefficient way of coping with the constantly changing nature and amount of work demanded. By using the more flexible types of contract listed above a Trust can vary the size and nature of its skills base or 'switch on' and 'switch off' elements of the workforce to match contractual changes. Balancing temporary contract workers, bank workers and permanent staff in such a mixed economy can, however, create problems of continuity and of cohesive team working.

This policy also has obvious consequences for the employee. It means less security of employment and a less easily predicted career structure. It also means employees must increasingly be willing to be flexible, move geographically, transfer their skills or retrain to meet changing employer demand.

From the employer's viewpoint flexibility is a key variable which means almost all contingencies can be managed without necessarily having planned for them. However, such flexibility does work both ways and Trusts without a sufficient core workforce may find that they lack the capacity to deliver quality work.

Supply

Since the passing of the National Health Service and Community Care Act 1990 several major changes have taken place nationally in the health labour market and in the way labour is utilized by Trusts. By their nature these changes affect career opportunities and employment policies.

The most significant change, perhaps that which has formed the basis of the others, is the large number of prospective employees who have training but no employment. For the foreseeable future in the acute, if not community sector, there will be more people available for work than there will be work places for them. Much professional training has transferred to universities from the old District Health Authorities so students are no longer employees. In the medium term these universities are over-providing trained health professionals in many areas as new educational contracts adjust to Trusts' employment fore-casts. Amongst the students or newly-qualified this means failure in their job search or doing something other than that which they have trained for, surrender of personal goals and loss of motivation. For individual Trusts the general over-supply means a large pool of candidates for many jobs but also candi-dates who are not suitable due to lack of recent experience.

The supply picture is by no means consistent. In certain specific areas, locations and specialities supply does not exceed demand and managers need to assess their own local situation for the staff they employ. The education providers need to consider the service impact of having programmes which are difficult to access when the skill is in short supply.

Returners

The health service has a predominately female and professional workforce. The training for many health service occupations is counted in years and highly skilled and expensive. The high proportion of women means the age profile of health service employees typically shows a dip between the mid-twenties to mid-thirties. Employees typically give five years service after qualification, then leave sometimes for a year or for longer. Trusts cannot simply rely on the newly qualified out-turn from the education providers each year for their new vacancies and the health service cannot afford to get such a short productive life from highly trained staff. One objective of those planning services should be to see the age profile of their employees recover as close to the level prior to the dip as possible or to prevent that dip altogether.

In practical terms the objective is to see the eventual return of as high a proportion as possible of the leavers aged in their twenties and thirties to the service or to their profession. Further it is to put in place policies so that as few as possible feel that to have children they have to break their employment.

Some policies which enable staff to continue in productive employment include:

- crêche facilities,
- term-time only employment contracts,
- flexible working hours,

- holiday play schemes, and
- paternity leave.

The policies which enable employees who have taken a break to return are:

- career break schemes,
- job share schemes,
- part-time options to return,
- return to work training or update,
- child-minder registers, and
- bank employment.

Many managers currently hold a view that if staff wish to go over to part-time status then they should return on a lower grade; this signals that returners are 'second class' and puts many off returning. As most people in this category are women, showing less favourable treatment in this manner is probably indirect discrimination and so unlawful. Another problem often faced is children's illness or a failure of child-minding cover causing the employee to need time off with no honest facility for taking that time. An extension of the use of what health service managers know as 'compassionate leave' to allow for an occasional domestic crisis may be appropriate. Given the nature of the health service and its workforce it may pay a Trust to develop more 'family-friendly' employment practices.

The manager in making manpower plans needs to consider the proportion of the work population of the appropriate age who may be permanently or temporarily out of paid employment and of those who leave how many can be counted as potential employees who may return in the future.

Assumptions that women returners are more likely to have absences from work, have poor time-keeping or leave more readily should not be made and are not valid. Indeed, the continued presence of such false assumptions often causes the more forward-thinking services to keep the gender, marital status or age of candidates from any shortlisting process.

Planned reduction

Plans like those described above may suggest to a manager that the organization needs to reduce its employed headcount over a period of time (as in Table 3.2).

In such a case investigations should be conducted concerning the internal organization; such as numbers and types of skills employed, typical turnover levels, retirements due, numbers of temporary contracts and numbers of casual staff.

Although an overall reduction might be forecast some sections or skills may need to expand or form a greater part of the new whole and so the skills required may be in short supply or secure. In this situation a succession plan should be considered as part of the overall plan.

It is important for managers in planning staff reductions to try to avoid any need for compulsory redundancy. Turnover and retirement rates will, as described, form a set of naturally occurring leavers in any time period. If this loss in numerical terms equals the overall reduction sought life is easier for the manager but the problem is not solved. Leavers may not come from the areas that need the reduction and so staff may need to be retrained and redeployed. In some cases leavers simply have to be replaced through external recruitment despite the overall down-sizing.

If such a balance of leavers and planned reductions is not to be arrived at naturally a voluntary early retirement scheme could be considered to encourage more leavers and so bridge the gap; this is explored in more detail from p 58 onwards.

The department or Trust may let staff know the forecasts and the problems faced and so allow employees to seek employment elsewhere, again increasing the number of leavers. Liaison with similar departments in other Trusts in the same location may enable them to fill their vacancies from the reducing workforce so avoiding the need for redundancy.

If natural wastage, retirement, early retirement and assisted transfer, alongside recruitment control, cannot achieve the required reduction in the time span necessary redundancy has to be considered. Using a forecasting model of predicted leavers it should be possible to determine how many redundancies may be required. Voluntary redundancy may be offered before any selection criteria regarding compulsory redundancy are arrived at through the necessary consultation.

Redundancy

As services change in their style and distribution so, as described, there may be consequences for staff employed. Increasingly the health market requires employers and staff to acknowledge a climate in which both must embrace and continually adapt to change. This means encouraging staff to be flexible in the nature of the work they carry out and the location of that work. If staff and employers are flexible and creative, redundancy can often be avoided.

'Redundancy' has the meaning given to it by the Employment Protection (Consolidation) Act 1978, section 81(2) and (3). Redundancy is the situation an employee faces when:

- the employer has ceased, or intends to cease, to carry on the business for the purposes for which the employee was engaged; or

- the requirement of the employer to carry out work of a particular kind in the place where staff are employed has ceased or diminished.

Statutory minimum periods of consultation exist. If the number of staff at risk of redundancy is between 10 and 99 then consultation with the staff and their representatives with a view to reaching some agreement should extend for at least 30 days prior to any decision. If 100 or more employees are involved the period is at least three months.

As has been seen various measures can be taken to avoid compulsory redundancy including:

- natural wastage,
- straightforward transfer to other work,
- redeployment to a suitable alternative,
- ending temporary employment,
- retirement because of organizational change, and
- voluntary redundancy.

If such measures to avoid compulsory redundancy fail then the consultation with individuals and their representatives will need to include general discussion of the required number of job losses and the criteria by which staff will be selected for redundancy. Considerations for specific discussion with individual members of staff will include:

- pension entitlements,
- redundancy compensation,

- periods of notice, and
- time off to seek alternative work.

The advantage of advance planning is that recruitment can be controlled so that when situations become vacant they either remain vacant or can be filled internally using the at-risk employees as an internal market. External recruitment can be restricted or stopped.

Redeployment

If a reduction in the size of the workforce is planned well enough in advance the opportunity for the organized redistribution of excess labour is much greater. A tendency towards annual purchasing contracts or 'one-off' initiatives makes planning difficult within the short-term time horizon.

The manager should see the employees at risk of redundancy at the earliest opportunity to discover their capacity to be redeployed to alternative work, including:

- skills used or available,
- location or ability to travel,
- hours of work,
- experience,
- types of work which would be considered as suitable, and
- willingness to change or consider alternatives.

An employee is not redundant if a suitable alternative employment opportunity exists with the same employer. In these circumstances dismissal on the grounds of redundancy would be classed as unfair and could give rise to a claim. At the same time if employees reject an offer of suitable alternative employment without good reason then they are not redundant and so employment can be terminated without a redundancy payment. Figure 3.1 shows a typical redundancy management programme involving a combination of seeking volunteers and redeployment to existing vacancies to avoid compulsory redundancy.

Early retirement

The main benefit to a Trust in offering early retirement is that it can avoid redundancy. Early retirement can clear career

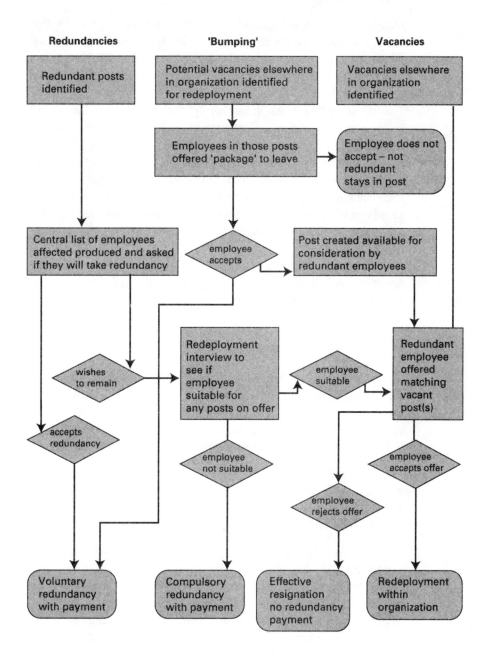

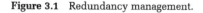

Figure 3.1 Redundancy management.

channels from the top end to allow progression within the organization. Those who wish to retire and have been looking forward to the opportunity can take that option. These advantages may convince the manager of the wisdom of an early retirement policy.

Such a policy does, however, place a long-term financial burden on departments. Very capable employees with valuable knowledge and experience may be lost and the age profile damaged. The department may be left with a less experienced workforce at a time when it may require its longer serving experienced employees the most. The superannuation scheme provisions mean it is seldom financially possible for the employer to facilitate an early retirement unless the post is redundant.

Pre-retirement preparation would seem to be essential to assist employees into early retirement resulting from organizational change or redundancy.

Diagnosis

So far workforce information has been suggested as a tool for forward planning purposes. It is also possible to use the same data to indicate the state of the current workforce and how it could be different in the future.

Examples of the kind of workforce data which act as an indicator are:

- staff absence rates,
- staff turnover,
- stability rates,
- overtime levels,
- workload produced, and
- vacancy levels.

Figures on staff absence will include annual leave, sickness, compassionate leave, maternity leave, public holidays, study leave and so on. Each represents a loss of productive staff time which may or may not be acceptable depending on its type and level. If uncertificated sickness absence in a particular group of staff is in itself too high to sustain an efficient business operation or if it compares unfavourably with other similar groups of staff then management action will be necessary.

The raw data is simply an indicator of a problem and does not provide an explanation for the feature it records. Further investigation will be necessary to see why a group highlighted works more overtime than other groups, has more sickness absence or suffers a higher level of leavers. Finding the cause or managing the symptoms may both of themselves change the behaviour of the group in the future. Having set appropriate trigger levels to stimulate further examination, managers may want to get down to the level of the individual and see, for example, those employees who have had more than ten days sickness absence in the last twelve months, or teams with more than £3 000 in overtime earnings over a set period.

Having a reliable set of data about staff allows management by exception, bringing individuals or groups which lie outside the normal parameters to the attention of managers. However, achieving this type of management does require regular access to and monitoring of statistical data by those managers.

Summary

In this chapter the issues covered have been the place of people in business planning, information requirements and technology to support those requirements. Then simple demand and supply plans were described. Given such plans exist the chapter finally looked at how the human resource might be managed in a way which makes it more flexible to meet business plans. Finally, given that a database exists, the use of that data to manage the current workforce was explored.

References

Mathis, R.L. & Jackson, J.H. (1988), *Personnel/Human Resource Management*. 5th Edn. West Publishing Company.

Further information

Institute of Employment Studies
University of Sussex
Falmer
Brighton
Sussex
BN1 9RF   (01273) 686751

Chapter 4:
ORGANIZATIONAL
STRUCTURE

Introduction

The imposition of an orderly structure to the undertaking of any complex task is essential, especially so when the activity undertaken relies on many different people each making a contribution. Organization is critical to success. That organization can be logistical, structural or procedural. This chapter is primarily concerned not with the work organization of individual employees but with the structural design of health service organizations against issues of management control, clinical autonomy and specialization. It aims to assist managers in analysing, designing and maintaining an effective organization or team. Managers have choices about structure and organization, they can, among other options:

- allocate tasks and responsibilities,
- designate reporting relationships,
- group individuals into work teams,
- delegate authority, or
- change job content.

The nature of formal structures will be examined and types of structures explored alongside the participant's individual roles.

Learning outcomes

- To understand the characteristics of traditional formal structures of organization.

- To perceive that underneath the explicit formal structure of an organization a complex informal set of interactions exists.

- To understand some of the cultural differences between health professionals and how organizational structure can reinforce those differences.

- To be aware of some of the fundamental structural choices that exist in designing health services.

- To gain an appreciation of the place of clinical directorates as a structural feature of health organizations.

Formal structure

Structures can be explicit and described in a formal way in an attempt to regulate the relationships between people at work. These formal structures are often created in the health service as bureaucracies in the traditional sense i.e. people report to each other in a command and control (or master and servant) relationship, each having a relative seniority with lines that can be drawn to describe those links. Classical bureaucracies were originally described by Weber (1947) and they remain, despite time and fashion, the predominant way of structuring public organizations. Weber's bureaucracy held all the features of today's health service including task division, hierarchy, rules, procedures and the concept of posts existing separately from the person holding the post. The Whitley job grading system in the main reinforces the hierarchy or seniority by describing each professional group's rank in a technical or management ladder.

Such formal structures often appear as pyramids but historically in the health service it looked more like a box structure as each specialization had its own complete and separate career structure to the top, as illustrated in Figure 4.1(a). The top team historically managed as equal individuals with decisions based on consensus. Much has happened in the last fifteen years to narrow the numbers at the apex of this organizational pyramid using general managers and more recently clinical directors, as illustrated in Figure 4.1(b).

Bureaucratic structures require that, if the number of staff completing a task is between five and ten, then depending on its nature a more senior 'span-breaker' is required in the structure to co-ordinate them. This tends to create layers of seniority and so middle-managers and supervisors. Another reason to create layers of seniority is increasing task complexity requiring problems to be 'delegated' up a competence ladder.

Peculiar difficulties exist in the health service in trying to describe the organizational structures on paper as a

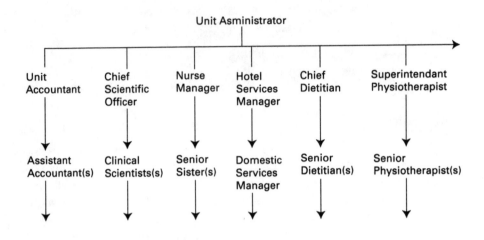

Fig. 4.1(a) Professional structure.

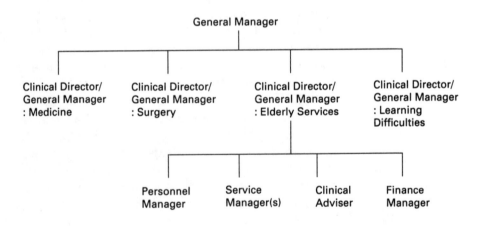

Fig. 4.1(b) General management structure.

bureaucracy. Each professional group has its own history, culture, role and statutory basis. The concept that a manager from one profession can or should manage another does not have automatic legitimacy. However, putting aside that specific problem health service hierarchy can ordinarily be clearly presented in structure charts on paper so that each person knows the job they are in, its place in the structure and the place of others. This can be seen in Figure 4.2.

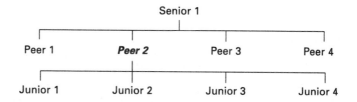

Fig. 4.2 Bureaucratic structure.

It is important to examine carefully the number of layers of hierarchy between the chief executive and the patient. The flatter the structure the closer decision-making is to the patient and the more efficient the work processes.

Bureaucracy has a price which is easy to demonstrate. A span of control set for each supervisor typically managing five direct subordinates means a workforce of 500 staff will need 100 first-line supervisors, 20 second-line and four third-line managers reporting to the ultimate manager. So the original 500 have an automatic management cost of 125 line reports regardless of need. Increasing the number of reports in any span of control to ten before allowing a supervisor means the 500 have only 56 line managers and one less layer in the hierarchy.

Activity

Count the numbers in the spans of control in your own structure charts and observe their effect on the layers of management required.

Ideal spans of control depend on:

- the manager's ability to delegate tasks,
- the amount of necessary personal contact,
- the subordinates' ability to motivate and manage them-selves,
- the amount of feedback required, and
- the management style adopted.

The culture of an organization can empower people to be creative or it can define and restrict individual freedom to act.

Excessive insistence on authority and having power centralized in key roles, rather than shared, restricts the potential for managers to expand their spans of control.

Grade drift

Although good spans of control may have been achieved before introducing a span-breaker, time and human behaviour can corrupt the new efficiency. Given a structure where they are receiving ten direct reports managers may see an available 'grade space' between themselves and their ten reports and seek to upgrade one of the reports to a more senior position so as to fill the perceived gap. This is illustrated in Table 4.1 below.

Table 4.1 Corruption of spans

Grade	Original	Corruption	Function
Grade 4	1	1	(receiving reports from Grade below
Grade 3	0	1	(receiving reports from Grade below reporting to Grade above)
Grade 2	10	9	(productive)

In creating this new one-to-one reporting relationship between the more senior report and themselves and removing themselves from the direct reports of the other nine the managers:

- add one layer to the hierarchy,
- remove an otherwise productive member of staff from the line,
- add to pay costs, and
- may make themselves effectively redundant.

The patient, in these bureaucratic games, falls to the bottom! Staff with experience or competence rise in the structure and lose contact with patients. This organizational design is good for neither the patient nor the health service. In representational terms the patient has no seniority or status. More recently these structures have been drawn upside down with the patient at the top and each layer below that seen as supporting the front-line staff. Although a gimmick, it does imply a different message about the organization's thinking.

The original concept of the nurse clinical grading structure was to allow nurses to progress in their clinical expertise without losing contact with patients or patient care. Progression did not, in theory, depend on rising within the management bureaucracy but in practice clinical grades G, H and I were used for nurse managers who had very little contact with patients.

Informal structure

Descriptions of the formal structure of an organization tend to talk about jobs, teams and structure without considering the real people and personalities that occupy those roles. The individual people and their formal roles in the workplace are inseparable issues and one factor impacts on the other. Whether the organizational design is driven by the people with the required skills or the formal structure (and which is more appropriate) makes for healthy debate.

The lines on organizational charts often do not reflect the reality or complexity of the real communication lines between people within work groups. Alliances, friendships and sources of information make the drawn organizational chart seem simplistic.

It is the people who make otherwise difficult organizational arrangements work successfully. Managers who have to co-ordinate and integrate the work and priorities of different senior professionals succeed not because of their positional authority but because of their personality. Producing a structure chart showing a line of accountability is guaranteed to fail in a group of health professionals who each perceive that they have clinical autonomy. Professionals see their profession as the source of authority and within multi-disciplinary teams the individual professionals see themselves as islands, each having monopoly and autonomy in their own field.

Different health care professionals find it difficult to work as a patient-focused team because:

● they are not organized structurally within the system to work together;

- they reach their professional status through independent routes with little stress on interdependency;
- the content of their training does not suggest shared values or methods of working but provides unique group identities;
- differences in perceptions of status or importance create tensions, reinforced by reward structures; and
- moves toward removing the lines of demarcation can be seen as threatening to some and leads to a creation of territorial feelings.

Managers in attempting to design seamless working teams and structures which involve each making their contribution in collaboration with others need to respect the diversity of the team. However, each does have a common interest or goal which brings them together and that should be the source of their unity.

The most appropriate organizational structure is the one that enables the organization to deliver its strategic intentions. In the health service this means structures should be created with the intention they have a five year life. The inappropriateness of a Trust's organizational structure may be an index of its ability, or lack of it, to move forwards the human aspect of strategy.

Power and professionals

Each professional group represents a power base with its own interests and ideologies. Griffiths (1983), in recommending the introduction of general management to the NHS, did recognize the problem of having competing bases of power but did not solve it. The introduction of general managers did not consolidate but simply added one more team into the play for power and for the control of resources.

It was said by Leo Tolstoy in *War and Peace* that 'if many simultaneously and variously directed forces act on a given body, the direction of its motion cannot coincide with any of those forces'. For example, imagine a circle of people of various physiques pushing a ball with none able to predict the ball's actual direction of travel. For this reason decision-making in the health service tends to be resultant or emergent rather than rational. General management was an attempt to create a single force and so a clear and single direction. The actuality was not as originally intended.

The problem of managing health services cannot be ignored. Managers have to try to create structure and organization. The question 'Why?' may be asked but, as Isaac Newton put it in his first law of motion, a body at rest will tend to remain at rest unless acted upon by an *external* force. Be warned, however, according to Newton's third law every action has an equal and opposite reaction.

So who is really in charge?

- The doctors, in their role as directors of care, simply because their clinical autonomy is privileged and it is they who commit and consume resources.

- The managers (and the Trust Board on whose behalf they act) in order to meet their statutory duties. As a 'quango' a presumption may exist that the Trust Board is accountable and so in charge.

- The purchasing authorities and fundholding general practitioners – 'he who pays the piper calls the tune'.

- The NHS Executive and its outposts, as the health service is a national public service.

- The politicians, in their duty to the public for a public service.

- The patients, as everything is done in their name.

The answer may still be that, in such a complex framework, no-one is actually nor ever can be in charge. All players do still negotiate with the others. The aim must be, therefore, to ensure that each group within a Trust or sub-division of it takes some ownership of or interest in its management.

Two examples of the management dilemma

Doctors

Medical staff can often seem not to accept the legitimacy of other health professions or alternatively appear to see them as subordinate to medicine. The ability of many doctors to undertake private work gives them a different sense of loyalty toward their hospital employers, although others have a greater vested interest in their departments being successful. The rotational nature of medical training between different hospitals, means loyalty to the organization is often lacking and the goals of the individual doctor have primacy. It is, therefore, difficult to tie doctors into the organizational structure, to have them accept the influence of others or to participate in management processes. There is still a belief amongst some medical staff that the work will be there for them whether the host organization manages its affairs well or not. This can lead to some opting out of the role bestowed upon them to participate in management. As a group the consultant body is very powerful at all levels of the health service and can exercise that power to protect individuals in the group at the cost of other's careers.

As the health service was conceived to provide free access to health care regardless of ability to pay, medical staff thought themselves free to pursue the good health of those in their care without constraint. But even at the beginning Aneurin Bevan warned that doctors should have a greater regard to the financial constraints on the service within which they work. Medical staff need to understand that their activities cost money but create measurable outputs and it is they who directly make the services efficient or inefficient. More than understanding the basic concept, doctors should be continually aware of the resources their activities consume against set budgets and, in partnership with their professional colleagues, be seeking to maximize their productive activities in relation to the contracts obtained by the organization.

To harness key components of the health care team, clinicians should be involved in management decision-making. The careful balance to be struck here is keeping medical staff involved in management while also leaving them free to do what they do best, making their unique clinical contribution, and having professional managers to do the managing.

Nurses

Nurses in the pre-Griffiths health service maintained their own independent management structure to which only nurses had access. It was not considered legitimate for nurses to be managed except by themselves. It often remains difficult for professional managers to manage nurses without this becoming an issue for those being managed. Indeed, many non-nursing managers find it necessary to designate an immediate report as their nurse adviser in order to compensate for their perceived lack of professional knowledge or a necessary qualification. The advantage for nurses of the new structures is that they can now choose a clinical or managerial career route, and the managerial route gives access to managerial positions which extend beyond managing nurses.

An effective source of nursing advice is important for managers, whether or not they originally qualified as nurses, as clinical nurses have a perspective on the patients and care standards which should be heard in decision-making. The designation of a post such as that of nurse adviser may be the structural way of achieving the input needed. This thinking clearly lies behind the decision to demand that Trust Boards contain an executive who is a nurse.

Activity

Locate yourself on your structure chart and decide whether the care professionals you formally manage in this structure really do recognize and own your agenda.

Structural choices

Managers have options on how to structure their organization, whether that be as a loose group of independent individuals or in a more formal way. In looking at the structure charts of different Trusts (or if historical structure charts are examined) it is possible to see each of the options in operation. The options reflect choices about what should drive the organization.

Functional structure

The first option is to divide the organization into its constituent functions. That is that finance, planning, contracts, personnel and patient care (often called operations) are separately designated and form reports to the chief executive or unit general manager. The rest of the organization follows those particular 'fault lines' so that each management function remains autonomous of the others right through to the patient. The obvious disadvantage of this option is that the staff functions dominate the agenda to the detriment of patient care issues.

Professional structure

A second option is to divide the organization by the major professional groupings. The requirement for Trusts to have executive directors named as the medical and nursing directors, and the formation of the Whitley Council groups into professional groups, suggests this option very strongly. The team would consist of Nursing, Medical, Professional, Technical and Support Service Managers. This option has its own history and known difficulties given that the patient is cared for by a multi-disciplinary team. Having the professional dominate does not necessarily provide for a customer focus.

Market structure

The third option is to divide the organization by customer or geography. So the Trust has Host Purchaser, Fundholding and Other Purchaser service heads. An alternative is a geographical differentiation by locality. This has the advantage of enabling management of the needs of particular customer groups but it does fragment or share the otherwise coherent management of particular facilities, services or resources between customer groupings.

Clinical structure

A fourth option is to manage by clinical grouping or product e.g. client or patient groups like Women's and Children's Services, Medical Services, Surgical Services, Head and Neck, Learning Disabilities, Elderly or whatever is appropriate. This kind of multi-divisional differentiation does allow management integration within each division.

Mixing the options

The choice of primary denominator does not have to remain as the structure descends. For example, if the primary denominator for the top team is function, they may then decide that clinical or product divisions should report to them and the structure within each clinical division may be on a professional basis. What is important is that, given the needs of the organization, all managers give conscious thought to and make explicit the structural characteristics they wish to see. The decisions will impact on the distribution of power, the content of the organization's agenda and its style of operation.

Activity

Which structure does your organization utilize and which should it utilize?

	Present	Desired
Functional	☐	☐
Professional	☐	☐
Market	☐	☐
Clinical	☐	☐

Clinical directorates

The present trend within Acute Care Trusts is to redesign the organization into a divisional structure based on clinical groupings of services. The primacy of the clinical group is being reinforced by the appointment of a lead clinician or clinical director to head that division. This has clear advantages to Trust Boards. Such a structure allows maximum decentralization to the divisions which internally integrate the other management and support functions. This makes the pricing of contracts, the measurement of performance and disinvestment of less successful individual parts of the organization much easier. The clinical directorate structure allows the potential for involving doctors in management, bringing decisions closer to the patient, creating multi-disciplinary working with particular patient groups and a diversity of approach.

At the same time, however, management and control become more complex. What starts off as clinical diversity can become goal diversity.

Centralization or devolvement

Nationally the tendency in the public sector and beyond is to decentralize or disaggregate large organizations into smaller units. The health service, as explored in Chapter 1, is also undertaking a decentralization of control and decision-making. Nationally the tendency is to devolve from head office structures to 'plant' level but Trusts as 'plants' are also taking this principle into their internal structures.

This is expressed in the movement toward the creation of clinical directorates which takes the trend to devolution to the internal structure of individual NHS Trusts. Trust Boards become a parent to a federated group of semi-autonomous organizations.

A centralized structure helps managers to act together within a whole organization perspective. Control and direction is readily achievable with some sense of consistency. In a decentralized structure it is more difficult to manage, internal competition replaces corporacy and communication is less effective across the organization. A potential for duplication exists and each decentralized unit requires more management time and resources.

Decentralization does make an organization's agenda more patient orientated; it also enables quicker decision-making and better reaction to specific or local events. Senior managers at the centre can be freed from more routine matters to concentrate on strategy. The problems of centralized control and its cumbersome character are avoided.

In its implementation decentralization does carry with it difficulties. NHS Trusts are often loathe to be explicit about what has been devolved to directorates and what has not. The model of a holding company and its sub-divisions does not suffice. Holding companies manage their divisions through a few key indicators such as return on capital employed. Trust Boards as statutory bodies (and their managers) will not give directorates that level of freedom. The result tends to be operational empowerment of directorates while the Trust makes strategic choices and maintains regulatory controls to limit the discretion of directorates and so ensure the accountability of the Trust as a whole.

Role and responsibilities in a directorate structure

As its centre the Trust Board discontinues its operational concerns and with this freedom takes up a role which can feature:

- appointment to key positions,
- strategic direction planning,
- policy formulation,
- monitoring and control,
- managing external relationships,
- integrating different activities,
- resource allocation, and
- intervention when necessary.

The directorates for their part have a semi-autonomous role in:

- meeting targets set by the Trust,
- implementing Trust policy,
- meeting service contracts,
- managing delivery of services, and
- ensuring economy, efficiency and effectiveness.

Clinical directorates are handicapped or incomplete if large parts of the organization remain functionally or geographically structured. To be effective the sub-divisions of an organization need to be integral or complete in themselves. In a sense the structure within the clinical directorate should be a replica of the Trust's structure. So in principle operational support services like finance, personnel, hotel services etc., should be divided and devolved so far as possible to the clinical directorates so an integrated team approach to the delivery of health care is possible. Certain corporate functions will require to remain central and form part of the 'core' of the Trust. The devolution choices for non-clinical services would seem to be:

- retaining a central service which enters into service or performance agreements with the clinical directorates concerning its standards, contribution, accessibility and responsiveness;

- linking the service to a particular clinical directorate which provides that service on behalf of or for the others on an internal trading basis;

- having the central service devolve its budget and so become a trading organization with each clinical directorate; or

- devolving the staff, budget and responsibility to the clinical directorates.

The small core of services left in the centre are often required to set up project teams on specific issues using clinical directorate staff, as the centre should find it lacks the necessary skills at this level following devolution.

Managing devolved structures without direct line authority is more difficult. The options which remain available for control are:

- target setting and monitoring,
- management by objectives,
- specifications or contractual agreements, or
- shared vision and values.

Change

Organizational structure in the health service constantly changes and is driven by diverse factors such as political imperative, a change of senior management, problems which associate themselves with existing ways of organizing and now market forces. Staff in the health service are very familiar with what can be perceived as 'management reshuffles'. The problem with this reality is that no one structure has a realistic chance of settling; managers can find themselves constantly in an induction crisis. However, the kind of chaos created by organizational change can have benefits in bringing forward new people, finding new opportunities, creating flexibility and blowing away cobwebs (in whichever form they take).

It would be better for one structure to be tried, tested and evaluated before decisions are made about its future and for changes to be seen as improvements rather than changes for the sake of change itself. Clinical directorates will have their day and will, hopefully, provide their own lessons in the design of health services.

Summary

This chapter explored traditional ways of describing and viewing organization. Then some of the issues specific to health services were examined, including the role of professionals such as doctors and nurses. Some structural choices were offered for consideration and clinical directorates explored alongside the issue of management devolution.

Recommended further reading

Handy, C. (1993) *Understanding Organisations*, 4th Edn., published by Penguin Books.

References

Griffiths, R. (1983) *NHS Management Enquiry: Letter to Secretary of State for Social Services from R. Griffiths (Leader of the Enquiry) (The Griffiths Report)*. HMSO, London.

Weber, M. (1947) *The Theory of Social and Economic Organisation*, Free Press, Glencoe.

Chapter 5:
LABOUR UTILIZATION

Introduction

Hospitals and community health service Trusts are large employers, often the largest employers in the locality. Health services need large numbers of people, they need a wide range of skills and rely on the people with those skills to provide the care for which the national service is known. The people employed in health care in such numbers need to be utilized properly to maximize the advantage to be gained from their skills. As money for health care, through contract, is limited and demand for care exceeds the cash limits, no money should be spent unless it:

- increases the quantity of care,
- increases the quality of care, or
- directly supports the infrastructure of care provision leading to the above.

Davies (1957) identified the need for 'a determination of the means of establishing a minimum economic cost or a maximum economic productivity criterion'. While the service relies on its people it is not cost effective to pay staff to hold skills which are not needed or responsibility they do not exercise, or to employ more staff than is necessary. Staffing in a public service has to be appropriate to and sufficient for the task. In a new service or site it would be appropriate for managers to:-

- identify the set of tasks and processes to be undertaken,
- analyse the skills or competencies required to undertake those tasks, and
- design jobs or roles which contain the skills required,

before they employ the staff required.

This is possible, as will be seen later, only in a limited way within health, and generally because the services and jobs pre-exist any examination managers can only reprofile what is found. Nevertheless managers cannot make the assumption that the staff and skills presently available are those best suited to the task.

Scientific management

When Taylor (1947) began to write about his ideas in the early part of the 20th century the problem of achieving efficiency was a relatively new one. He considered the main obstacle to efficiency was a failure by managers to find ways to co-ordinate and control the workers and offer proper rewards for their co-operation.

He set out to devise methods of job study, control of work flow and incentives. His technical achievements are to be seen in present day time and motion studies, payment by results systems, production control systems, and so on.

For scientific managers the worker was a kind of mechanism who would, if given the right rewards, submit to being organized and manipulated to produce in pre-determined ways.

Taylor's ideas on human motivation are now seen as primitive, as he never understood the significance of groups in organizations. Organizations were seen as disorderly aggregates of individuals who were required by management to be drilled into formal order and given direction by formal structure, procedure and control.

The six faces to labour utilization

This chapter will examine six aspects of efficient labour utilization and then describe, in some detail, two processes to ensure it. The six aspects considered in detail below are:

- labour substitution,
- staff numbers,
- skill-mix,
- grade mix,
- labour flexibility, and
- role restriction.

As will be seen when the processes are described in the next section, to ensure best utilization of labour the aspects considered below cannot be seen separately in analysis. It is, however, useful to deal with them separately as an introduction to the processes themselves.

Labour substitution

In the health service labour is a factor of production, alongside land, capital and enterprise. The cost of running any particular health service is distributed across these four factors. The ideal mix will produce a quality service at the lowest cost. Each factor, including labour, has a cost and a level of efficiency which can be measured. If the price of the labour employed rises it becomes relatively less efficient or reliable so it will be replaced by technology or alternative forms of labour.

In hospital Trusts this equation helps managers to determine whether capital and equipment should be organized to be available to the more expensive staff, or whether the staff should be organized to get the best from expensive capital assets. Also, this equation determines the balance of investment managers should make between labour and capital for their services. At the fringe this explains why the night catering service may come out of a vending machine!

Within clinical services, it may cost money to bring theatre staff in at night to run additional lists. More importantly, however, what is the opportunity cost of having expensive theatres lying idle for 12 hours in 24, missing waiting list initiatives? Clearly, in this example, the staff are organized to make full use of the capital asset. In the same way, but a different answer this time, it costs money to run a pool of cars for community staff. Should the cars be kept running at all times, so a health visitor never waits for a car or are the car running costs so much that it is better occasionally for a health visitor to wait for one?

Activity

Think about the cost of the staff and capital you utilize to run your service. Decide which is the more expensive resource per unit used. Is your service provision labour or capital intensive? Given your answer, do you appropriately prioritize the way you run your service to maximize the use of the most expensive resources?

This aspect can be progressed through:

- management accounting,
- asset utilization surveys, and
- a work study.

It is not always appropriate for services to proclaim 'staff are our most valuable asset' as the economics may make it a false declaration.

Staff numbers

'Staff shortages' is a well-worn cry in health services and no doubt this reflects the difficulties that can be faced if numbers are set incorrectly. Numbers are inseparable from the efficiency of staff. A midwifery team will serve to illustrate the examination of labour efficiency purely in terms of numbers.

Case study – additional midwives

One midwife may look after two hundred or so women in the community and provide a standard service. If the caseload grows another midwife must be added to handle the increased work. With two they must now communicate with each other, cover for each other and keep records for each other's reference. The additional contribution made by having two midwives does not, therefore, double the caseload of the first.

When a third and fourth midwife are added to create a team against increasing workload the diminishing return from each becomes very evident. In addition to the reduced contribution from each, the real cost increases as the team demands structure.

One midwife must be responsible for clinical practice and teaching, another for management, so grades increase to reflect relative seniority. The larger the team the easier it becomes to add additional workers without seeing or indeed demanding additional outcomes at the original value. In fact, the team should only add additional staff until the cost of adding one more exceeds the income or quality benefit to be gained.

Unfortunately, many factors operate other than a wish to maintain maximum efficiency which means if two similar clinical services in different locations are compared their prices will vary as the labour component varies. If the quality of the service also varies in line with the higher staffing numbers and the local purchaser is willing to pay for that measurable quality difference then all remains well. If quality or quantity is not measurably different and purchasers are not prepared to pay or existing budgets are overstretched then operating with excess numbers cannot be justified.

If demand on the service is seasonal or care contracts are non-recurring (making work variable) then managers may seek flexibility in staff numbers employed to avoid short or excess staffing.

This issue can be progressed through:

- identification of core staffing requirements,
- recruitment,
- use of bank and agency staff,
- redeployment of staff, or
- redundancy.

Skill-mix

Many different professions operate within the health sector, some unique to health and some common to other industries. Each profession has its own history, skills, values, knowledge base and utility. Each also has a price. The wide range of skills and partnerships necessary to provide a health service makes it a complex but rich work environment. There is no simple link between skill of the labour input and the quality of the clinical output.

Some professions are obviously better suited to certain work processes than others. It is to the benefit of patients that managers seek to match patients' particular needs to the appropriate availability of specific skills at the right time. It is widely accepted, for example, that operating department practitioners have skills better suited to that environment and patients' needs at that time than nurses. The practitioners have specific training and utilize all their skills in that setting; nurses would require additional training, are more expensive and the manager would be paying for a wider set of skills they do not utilize. Health professionals should only be engaged in activities appropriate to the skills of each. Newman (1995), in examining house officers' job content, found that '80 percent of their time was spent clerking patients, form filling, chasing test results, finding x-rays, writing up patient charts and notes or portering samples and forms'. This represents a poor use of junior doctors' time.

As the various health professions tend towards post-qualification specialization into narrower roles, increase barriers to entry and increase their prices, so the incentive to replace them becomes greater. For example, the difference in price between a dietitian and a nurse with nutritional training is evident. Given junior doctors do twice the hours for the same pay as nurses, can nurses do more of what junior doctors do? Given a price difference the additional utility of the more expensive skills has to be clear if the skill-mix is to remain value for money. Getting the right skill-mix enables patients' varied needs to be met most economically by bringing together only the skills that are needed at a particular point in time.

This issue can be progressed through:

- cost benefit analysis,
- clinical audit, and
- training and development.

Grade mix

Within professions, levels of seniority exist dependent on technical or clinical expertise, responsibility carried or resources managed. If staff are required to have higher levels of technical competence, manage resources or to be held accountable then reward should follow. As with skill-mix, cost should not be incurred for expertise that will not be utilized, so higher grades within services need to be utilized to be justifiable.

Managers are under constant pressure from staff who think

their grades should rise and from market pressures which suggest they should fall. Ward managers, for example, will find this question arising when a nurse post becomes vacant. Professional nurses (Grade D under Whitley) are often new from college or university with a Project 2000 diploma or a degree in nursing. To employ this expertise costs more than employing a health care support worker, with a national vocational qualification in Care, who will be lower graded (Grade A under Whitley). While newly qualified professional nurses have a wider range of skills, for example they can assess and plan care, their immediate utility on the ward may be lower than that of the already proven practical competence of a support worker. The ward manager has a grade mix question and in part the answer depends on the mix of grades already in place and whether enough staff already exist with the planning, assessment and supervisory skills required. Similar questions about grade and seniority exist through the whole care structure.

Activity

Obtain a copy of, or draw, the existing structure chart for your team. Count the levels of different seniority or hierarchy between the patient and yourself. Ask yourself whether you know the unique added value provided by each level over that below it? Compare the structure of your service with a couple of others in your organization to see if different approaches are possible.

This issue can be progressed through:

- review of job descriptions against grading definitions,
- workforce planning,
- re-grading,
- protection of pay, or
- redeployment.

Labour flexibility

Managers can increase the utility of the labour they employ, and so improve the chances of those people remaining employable, by increasing flexibility. A more flexible worker is attractive as work based reaction time to patient needs is quicker and organizational change is possible without exposing employees to risk of redundancy.

To take an example, a porter is on a ward collecting a patient for an X-ray and the patient vomits, or spills a drink getting out of bed. Does the mess wait for a domestic assistant to come on shift, is a nurse pulled from her duties to clean up or does the porter attend to it? Can that same nurse or domestic put in a new lightbulb to the bedside lamp for the patient or does that take a visit from a maintenance assistant? Such demarcation lines are expensive, time wasting and they have an adverse effect on patients. Perhaps a new general worker is required to replace the existing roles of domestics, porters, catering assistants, housekeepers and ward clerks. Similar situations exist at the fringes of the nurse's role with those of doctors, physiotherapists, occupational therapists and so on. Nurses, for example, could undertake simple diagnostic tests and provide limited therapy.

Some roles have a core which is unique to that role and which may even have legal status, but much can be done to encourage flexible working at the margins of such roles to the benefit of patients.

The examples given above all concern an ability to deploy workers over a broader range of functional activities. This type of approach goes by various names; multi-skilling, job enlargement, generic working or functional flexibility. In the case of porters, domestics, ward clerks etc, this enlargement operates across a range of tasks at a similar level. Expanding the nurse's role to reduce junior doctors' working hours or the support worker's role to release skilled nursing time is enlargement of a different kind – expanding the ceiling of a post's ability to operate.

This issue can be progressed through:

- training and development,
- role enhancement,
- multi-skilling,
- removal of demarcation barriers, and
- empowerment.

Role restriction

While flexibility is crucial, to use the example above changing lightbulbs should not be a part of a trained nurse's regular duties. Certain skills have a premium attached to them so that they are expensive to buy. If the person with those skills works within a system which routinely takes them away for a significant time from utilizing their core skills then money is being wasted. For example, to see managers photocopying or trying to arrange meetings, trained nurses serving patients drinks or doctors filing patients' notes as a routine part of what they each do is not a cost effective way of working. If support workers are allowed to expand their ability to operate, those in the supported role have more time to do what they are trained and paid for.

This issue can be progressed through:

- job descriptions,
- work organization, and
- management study.

Two processes for critical observation

A dangerous presumption can be made at this point that what health service organizations need is fewer employees, less qualified and 'jacks' rather than 'masters'. More appropriately, managers should be prompted to examine critically the labour utilization within their service. The following two processes are aimed to break the status quo or the presumption all is well. They are intended to get managers and staff to think again about staffing. Both processes start with the work to be done, from different standpoints, and proceed back to the staffing requirement. The very fact that the processes begin with the work to be done means the result will not match the existing situation. Reviews of this kind are only successful if:

- change is intended,
- defensive behaviour is avoided, and
- authority exists to see the process through.

The commitment of those affected can be engaged if the reasons for the process are clearly explained and they are given an input or kept informed.

The processes examined are:

- process mapping, and
- reprofiling.

Process mapping

Many of the issues surrounding staff numbers, types and grades cannot be unravelled without analysing and changing work processes. The work processes which exist do so as a result of the staff resources deployed. Those processes may be over complex, unnecessary or fragmented, so taking up staff time or creating staff down-time unproductively. Processes are not designed to be inefficient, they typically have incrementally developed over time and expanded to fit the resources available. Often the process stays the same when the expected end result changes making the process inappropriate. The obvious way to start a critical examination of work processes is to focus on the individual patient (or typical patient) rather than start with existing work systems.

Step 1: Intervention planning

While in hospital or care the patient sees a variety of staff from across the disciplines, following a path through the system. Often the patient is the only common denominator between staff groups or departments. The first step is to bring together representatives of the different people who meet the typical patient. This will include a consultant, nurse, porter, receptionist or ward clerk, any relevant therapists and so on. Given the process outcomes usually cross departmental or professional boundaries, the group will need a facilitator and authority to undertake its task.

Step 2: Investigation

The focus group described above will initially need to meet together to describe factually what they do at each stage of the patient's experience. If the patient arrives at reception first then what are the staff in contact with that patient doing at that time? By mapping the process beginning to end each member of the focus group has the opportunity to add their unique contribution. The process as it exists can then be recorded. While the staff involved work together every day (and so every day see the same patients as the others see) they will find the whole story surprising. Although they are the 'real' care team they will not have talked in this way. An extract from a typical process map which results from such an exercise is shown in Figure 5.1.

Patient activity	Organizational activity
Patient attends for appointment with Consultant	Clerk asks patient to fill in form
Patient returns form	Clerk receives the form Clerk logs patient arrival in book and checks availability of notes
Patient is weighed and measured	Nurse (I) weighs and measures patient Nurse (I) records data on routine card for medical notes Nurse (I) takes card and medical notes to Nurse (II)
Patient enters cubicle and undresses	Nurse (I) calls patient to cubicle and instructs to undress
Patient meets Consultant for first time	Consultant arrives and introduces self
Patient talks with Consultant and agrees treatment	Consultant conducts short interview examination, leading to recommendation of treatment

When nothing is recorded in the Patient activity column the patient is passive.

Fig. 5.1   Example of a process map.

Step 3: Critical analysis

Once the whole process is laid out on paper it becomes easy to see its problems. Delay, bureaucracy, ignored patient needs all come to light as the same focus group critically analyses their patient interventions. They as a team will start to raise questions about how co-ordination occurs, how communication is managed and how patients are dealt with. In the example in Figure 5.1, the consultant was meeting patients for the first time when the patient had been undressed and would be feeling ill at ease. The need for two nurses, and the content of their current role had to be questioned also.

Step 4: Design

Having identified problems with what exists it is a simple step to

move into work process redesign. This redesign will typically
raise issues concerning:

- staff levels e.g. unnecessary processes,
- roles e.g. the need for greater flexibility,
- structure e.g. bringing the 'real' team together,
- costs e.g. decentralization of decision-making and services,
  and
- quality e.g. improving the patient experience.

Staying with the same example, the process improvements
identified which might be produced by the group are shown
below.

(1) When the patient arrives for the first time at the front desk
they have a number of different needs which can be char-
acterised as:

- information i.e. what is going to happen today?
- reassurance i.e. what is going to happen to me?

Some of the patient's needs that are present do not appear
to be met by the current work process. 'Arrival' needs to
become as significant in the work process as it is for the
patient.

Suggested improvements:

- Health questionnaires or fact-sheets for new patients, to
  provide answers to common questions prior to first
  attendance.
- Address the patient's need for reassurance by finding a
  way of releasing existing nursing time to allow every
  new patient to be met by a nurse on arrival.

(2) When patients arrive they engage with an administrative
process which carries them through treatment. Some of
these processes are historically based and possibly dupli-
cate each other or existing hospital systems, and so are
unnecessary. These processes absorb large amounts of time
across team disciplines.

Suggested improvements:

- Abandon the current arrival book.

- Develop simplified patient administration.
- Review the need for the form given to the patient on arrival at reception.

(3) It was suggested by the group that, to speed up the clinic, patients were sometimes unaccompanied and inappropriately dressed when they first met the Consultant.

Suggested improvements:

- Devise and implement revised protocols for seeing patients.
- Examine the role of nurses in clinic (presently weighing, measuring and administration).
- Raise awareness of patient dignity.
- Examine average clinical appointment times to reduce over-running.

Paper based improvements will inevitably be naive but they do provide tests for the service.

Step 5: Implementation

Some of the actions required will be within the grasp of the focus group or care team and so implementation is achievable. Many issues will concern other parts of the service which impact on the focus group's patients. It is at this step that the value of getting clear commitment from the organization at large becomes so valuable. The frame of reference through which the focus group think about their work, each other and the patient will have significantly altered but they need to be empowered to turn their experience into reality.

The possible effect of running this project repeatedly across different areas of care is to:

- reduce the number and types of different staff a patient is transferred between;
- bring facilities and services closer to the patient;
- develop care protocols and schedules;
- reduce the amount of time patients spend in hospital or in care processes;
- reduce patient and staff delays;
- create multi-disciplinary care teams by devolving structures;

- integrate support services; and
- improve the patient's experience.

Reprofiling

The process described above can be very powerful if the team is cohesive, will put aside time to meet and are committed together to improving patient care. The members of the group, each from their own disciplines, need to be willing to self-examine their role critically and be open to change. Some services are not culturally set up to allow the approach set out above. Even given a meeting and a willingness to discuss the issues, the proposals produced by such a group are often excellent but, being self-generated, they are unlikely to place any of the team at significant risk. Reprofiling, as described below is a management process, which asks questions about the shape of the work team. The starting point for this process is not the individual or typical patient but the amalgamated workload as expressed in the contract for patient activity. Once a department or service has been selected the steps to follow are shown below.

Stage A: Data assimilation

The workload demands on a service may be expressed in a specific contract with a single host purchaser. This simple clarity is, however, increasingly less likely to exist. Several different contracts may be in place with a range of different purchasers and the service may be part of a block contract or at cost per case. Depending on the service selected, it may be based on a series of internal agreements rather than outside contracts e.g. theatres or pharmacy. A group is necessary which can identify and quantify the customer requirements: what is the work task? Later the group will need to be able to convert those work demands into process and resource implications. The group may include the service manager, a finance adviser, a personnel manager or workforce planner, a contracts manager and other more appropriate individuals with local expertise. This group, as can be observed, is distinctly different from a process mapping group.

As well as identifying customer requirements, as suggested above, the group may decide it needs some comparative data on the number, type and grade of staff utilized by other similar employers to produce similar activity levels.

Stage B: Task analysis

Having identified the work requirement, be it activity levels, price, quality standards, waiting times, contract monitoring information, the group needs to examine those facts critically and in sequence. Putting aside what happens now, the group needs to define what needs to be done (either directly or indirectly) to meet the requirements. For example, if a quarterly monitoring requirement exists, it must be decided what needs to be recorded, how it will be recorded, when it will happen, when the data will be consolidated and when presented to achieve the deadline. If a certain number of patients must be screened then consideration must be given as to how that happens: patients need inviting in, they need receiving, they need a bed, the bed needs sheets and so on. The appropriate task questions will be:

- What outcome is sought?
- What standards of care are expected?
- What activities meet that outcome?
- When do they need to happen?
- How do they need to happen in process terms?

The group may decide to categorize these activity sequence lists as, for example:

- clinical,
- hotel,
- administrative,
- technical, etc.

Stage C: Job analysis

Given a list of 'things to be done' this can be readily converted into lists of tasks. These tasks will fall into groups depending on the skill areas and the level of complexity. Such an analysis will suggest how many of what type of staff are needed.

Jobs can be defined from those groups of tasks, which will have been built up directly from necessary activities, to meet defined outcomes. The quantity of types of task in each category will determine job numbers and the level of task will determine grade mix.

The placing of tasks on a page creates the foundation for job descriptions. In some cases the content will dictate a traditional role, for example, assessing care needs may require a registered nurse or diagnosis a doctor. Other jobs may emerge which are new or at least a variant on what has been seen before. The job structure which results from such process will not bear much relation to the current structure. It is also important to be open minded, nurses might take a patient's history, refer a patient for tests or have a limited prescribing role.

Certain base principles may exist at the beginning of the job analysis, for example one registered general nurse at Grade D (Whitley) should be on each shift. Alternatively, comparative skill-mix data could be used to create a starting point if the blank page disturbs people in the team.

Stage D: Skills analysis

With a set of clear task based job descriptions it is then open to the group to produce personnel specifications or a skills map for the people required in the new posts. Partly this will aid recruitment and selection of future workers, mainly it will enable training needs to be identified for existing staff to meet the new roles. Many of the care competencies identified may be met through the new national vocational assessment structure.

Stage E: Planning

A personnel manager or workforce planner may be required if these skills are not already in the group at this stage.

A picture of the current staff is required so that this can be compared with the ideal position. Through selection, training, redeployment, natural wastage, redundancy, or other appropriate means over a period of time the old needs to be converted into the new. This clearly requires a plan which can be subject of consultation with the staff concerned in terms of content and timescale.

Stage F: Implementation

It is rare for the results of such fundamental reviews to be immediately actionable. A reasonable planned timescale will exist to install new roles, provide training and change standard practice. Given a clear end position, however, each opportunity presented, for example a staff vacancy, can be positively used to maintain the desired direction.

It is important to consult before the final picture (and the plan to reach it) becomes set. Such fundamental changes, if presented as a *fait accompli* or without explanation, may be resisted as a result of staff anxiety. The service needs to continue its work effectively during the change process and this requires co-operation from staff.

Focus on job analysis

Each of the labour utilization processes described above requires the participant managers to hold skills in job analysis. The job analysis tool is used to determine staff input required to satisfactorily perform a task or to determine the best method of utilizing staff to do that task. According to Davies (1966):

> 'Job design means specification of the contents, methods and relationships of jobs in order to satisfy technological and organisational requirements as well as the social and personal requirements of the postholder.'

The techniques used can include:

- questionnaires,
- observation,
- interviews with postholders,
- interviews with management, and
- creation of a task inventory.

Information is collected on:

- tasks done,
- skills needed,
- knowledge needed,
- responsibilities held,
- time involved, and
- methods employed.

Outcomes from job analysis

The outcomes that can be gained from such an analytical separation of job content are:

- information about which jobs should exist,
- a greater understanding of the relationship jobs should have to each other,
- details of what postholders are required to do,
- identification of the equipment and supplies necessary to do the job, and
- a definition of minimum skill requirements.

Consideration has to be given as to:

- why a job is done,
- what range of tasks is done,
- what the purpose is of each task, and
- how each task relates to the others.

Why reprofile?

People have a value to the organization in knowing it, working within it, developing specific skills and assisting in its success. As they will be an asset to future success, keeping such people and ensuring their productivity is obviously better than losing them. Likert (1967) said:

> 'These estimates of probable subsequent productivity, costs and earnings provide the basis for attaching to any profit centre, unit or total corporation a statement of the present value of its human organisation.'

Summary

The processes described for conducting a staff review are time consuming and complex. So why bother? The goals are obviously greater efficiency and value for money. The incentives are:

- to improve the likelihood of retaining existing contracts from purchasers,
- to enrich the job satisfaction of individual employees,
- to increase the price differential between the local and competitor services enough to attract new work,
- to have scope to re-invest labour cost savings from the service in new ways,
- to obviate the effect of present or future skills shortages,
- to compensate for the absence of Project 2000 students on academic studies,
- the ability to introduce flexible working or new working practices,
- the ability to recognize the real contribution made by the non-professional staff, and
- a possible reduction in junior doctors' hours.

Small changes in the margin are as, if not more, important than large scale reviews, in that actual change speaks louder than planned change. While considering the review processes contained in this chapter every vacancy should be seen as an opportunity to think again about the way in which work is done.

Recommended further reading

Further guidance is given by J. Bramham, *Practical Manpower Planning*, 3rd Edition (1982) produced by the Institute of Personnel Management.

References

Davies, L.E. (1957) Toward a theory of job design. *Journal of Industrial Engineering*, **8**, 19–23.

Davies, L.E. (1966) The Design of Jobs. *Industrial Relations*, **6**, 21–45.

Likert, R. (1967) *The Human Organisation: Its Management and Value.* McGraw-Hill Book Company, New York.

Newman, K. (1995) New Deal? Big Deal. *Health Service Journal*, **105**, 24–5.

Taylor, F.W. (1947) *Scientific Management.* Harper and Brothers, London.

Chapter 6:
REWARD

Overview

The money which a care provider receives is decided by the health contract negotiation process. Any staff expenditure has to be included in the price agreed.

Reward management and the internal market for health care are each new and unique parts of the latest reform of the health services. Each acts on the other to change its character. If providers of health care were held to fixed staff expenditure levels then price would not be a significant variable in choice of providers for care. If there were no internal market then no competitive pressure would exist for providers to manage their cost structures efficiently.

To sustain real increases in staff expenditure over inflation purchasers have to be persuaded they are getting more or better quality outcomes. Upward movements in staff expenditure can therefore only be accommodated by:

- reducing costs elsewhere,
- entering into debt,
- undertaking additional income-generating activities, or
- improving quality in a way that purchasers can measure and will fund.

Learning outcomes

- To realize the historical national context in which health managers have operated and the reasons for this model being rejected.

- To appreciate the opportunities and choices that Trust status offers to health organizations in regard to rewarding staff.
- To understand the factors which determine the level of reward appropriate to organizations, groups or individuals.

> ● To understand the difference between pay, benefits, terms and conditions and appreciate importance of each.

Freedoms

In *Working for Patients* (Department of Health 1989) it is stated in Chapter 3 that 'NHS Hospital Trusts will be free to continue to follow national pay agreements or to adopt partly or wholly different arrangements'. This intention of the government found its way into the National Health Service and Community Care Act 1990 at Schedule 16 which provides that:

> 'an NHS Trust shall have the power to do anything which appears to it to be necessary or expedient for the purposes of or in connection with the discharge of its functions including in particular the power to ... employ staff on such terms as the Trust thinks fit.'

Alongside the devolution of pay management to NHS Trusts, with statutory underpinning, the remaining directly managed units are finding that national arrangements are becoming more flexible. Local management of pay and reward is clearly part of today's health services management task. However, having the insight to see what can be done locally with the pay agenda and having the capacity to make those changes quickly are not the same thing.

The old constraints

Devolvement of pay management had been sought by health service managers for some time, but driven by dissatisfaction with the Whitley Council and Pay Review Body systems rather than by managers having any positive alternatives of their own. The central national system was perceived to be:

● bureaucratic,
● binding,
● inflexible,
● unresponsive, and
● over-regulating.

Personnel departments were interpreters of the rules and managers subject to those rules.

Haywood and Vinograd (1992) commented that 'because NHS pay has been determined centrally, Unit managers have previously had no reason or opportunity to take many major remuneration decisions. Complaints have frequently been made about having no significant control over some three-quarters of the total budget'.

When NHS Trusts were created the staff formerly employed by the District Health Authority previously, who transferred into the employment of Trusts, did so with their existing contracts of employment. The history of pay in the health service could not be left behind, rather it was imported wholesale with:

- uniform and rigid forms of work organization,
- fixed occupations,
- rigid job and grade categories,
- set working hours,
- dictated rates of payment,
- detailed terms and conditions of service.

All the above came into Trusts both in contracts of employment and in the minds of health workers. This was not only a problem inside the new health organizations but because each inherited the same package, which continued to operate nationally, it acted as a powerful benchmark from which every Trust started out.

The new opportunity

With the transfer of staff came the transfer of decision making. In the past Advance Letters 'arrived' to be implemented. The subject matter and content of such letters was determined by an outside body and they were written as instructions. There was no need or reason for hospital managers to think 'if I had to write the next one what would it be about?' When the opportunity for change came no-one in the new health organizations had the necessary experience, training or expertise in local pay determination.

Trusts had many new responsibilities and so the transition from directly managed unit to Trust and the first year as a Trust was often difficult. Reward management might have presented opportunities for future success but a usable system existed and so the subject did not require immediate attention. Many other issues came higher up the list of a new Trust's priorities such as:

- management structure,
- costing for contracting,
- identifying activity levels, and
- negotiating for income.

However, where new Trusts saw reward as a high priority it could be used pro-actively to change the world of work. The impact of introducing local pay flexibility at the same time as the internal market was to change the reward agenda within providers from a matter of unwelcome administrative control into a potential management tool.

What now?

Trusts as new entities have to set out their own long-term strategic direction taking account of:

- national policy on managing health and other national imperatives on managing staff (e.g. doctors' hours);
- relationships with purchasers;
- purchasers' plans for local health service delivery;
- the amount of business expected and how best to organize to provide care; and
- the clinical direction of care.

Such thinking leads on to thinking about the organization of work and rewards for work. Reward management cannot properly precede the wider considerations.

Having reached the stage of knowing what to do, why and to what end, the last hurdle is to take the transition from that which is given to that which is desired. Health managers have been accused of not making the most of their new pay freedoms, but perhaps in the light of the above it is instead surprising that so much has already happened and that so much is planned. Three immediate options exist, to:

- make a fresh start,
- move on from Whitley, or
- use existing flexibility within Whitley.

A fresh start

To bring plans into reality managers can choose to introduce the new arrangements on pay, terms and conditions for all new staff who join them from a fixed date. New staff can be recruited onto new contracts of employment from outside the NHS and so have no reference to or memory of anything different.

Disadvantages

Such new staff will talk to their work colleagues who will want to compare and contrast terms and conditions while they work alongside each other. If the new contracts are in some regards less favourable, then this will be seen by those on the old contracts as a future threat to their terms and by those on the new terms as unfair. If the new contracts are in some regard more favourable, then this will be seen by those holding old contracts, the long servers, as disloyal and may create a source of discomfort for staff enjoying the new terms.

Advantages

The advantage of this way forward is that it can be made clear to those who wish to retain their existing terms of employment that they can do so without any threat for the length of their employment, but the organization, given a steady rate of turnover, will in a decade move all its staff over to its own new terms independent of any national direction. The health organization which chooses this approach does however need to write its own terms as a founding package and needs to be able to operate that package alongside its myriad of imported Whitley Council conditions, always being aware whether any employee is 'local terms' or 'Whitley terms'. 'Red circling' or protecting the pay of those who remain on Whitley at a level above the new rates for the job may act as a defence to any equal pay claims from those on local terms.

Moving on from Whitley

Another approach is to seek to negotiate changes to the terms of employment of all existing staff, either with each individual staff member or with a body that has been formally recognized as acting for all staff. This approach is unlikely to create a great leap forward in the comparative sense but will move more people on to partially different terms more quickly. It is more difficult in this scenario to be reassuring because change is sought for all who will change, either directly or through their representatives. Existing staff are unlikely to agree to leave their contracts unless what is new looks to them to be more favourable. It may be that to make some changes which are considered critical to success, a trade off which the staff would find attractive is possible elsewhere in the package. Such winning combinations of changes can benefit the staff, the organization and the work, but are difficult to achieve in a complex organization.

Using existing flexibility

The last option open to managers is to speak where Whitley is silent and to determine locally where Whitley allows that flexibility. In this last example all the staff remain on or within national terms. The difficulty here is that:

- flexibility may be granted where it is not needed,
- it may not be granted where it is needed, and
- no adequate local framework will exist.

Activity

Think about which of the possible routes towards new arrangements would best suit your organization.

The need to change

In fact managers are using each of the above routes to change or else they have made a decision not to change away from Whitley so long as it exists to be administered. The no change option is being taken by very few considering the forces that exist making it the easiest and most attractive option in the short term.

Where is the imperative to do something that is both brave and different? A danger exists that if managers are not seen to be exercising their new freedoms false presumptions will be made about the lack of initiative or progress being shown and so those freedoms will be muted or eroded. Managers should see it as essential in the shorter term, while the political climate exists, to create irreversible divergence.

Work, or the way it is undertaken by people, can be distorted by the system used to reward it. Managers see around them a constant stimulus to change in the irritating work and pay practices which can be altered. Unsocial hours payments, overtime, on-call, stand-by and other allowances (worth so much on top of basic pay) create an incentive to obtain them whether earned or not. For example under Whitley terms, ancillary staff can roster themselves to work overtime then go on sickness absence with a continued entitlement to the enhanced payment while a colleague is called in from an off-day to cover! Another general effect is that Whitley rewards long service more than it rewards performance. Simply owning a desire to remove contrived work practices or to alter messages will lead to change to new reward systems.

The most powerful force for change is a realization that once the business has

- a direction of travel,
- a work load to tackle, and
- a best way of organizing to do that work

then pay can become an incentive to support appropriate behaviours. In this context reward management is about helping the achievement of objectives and so becomes central to the agenda rather than an adjunct to it. It takes some time to reach this point and reward must remain only one part of the overall policy structure with its place not overstated. Money is not the only motivator.

Lew Swift (1991) described the constraints thus:

'Local pay bargaining brings with it a great deal of flexibility; it is also accompanied by a number of powerful constraints. In particular, limitations will be imposed by the amount of finance available, determined policy and procedure, legislation and the need for a Trust to recruit and retain the right staff, maintain a good image and generally act in a prudent way.'

Despite those constraints local pay determination has a number of benefits:

- problems can be dealt with locally and quickly rather than waiting for a national compromise;
- the ability to implement or pay for decisions can be considered before the decision is made; and
- an honesty of approach has to develop when decisions have to be taken locally rather than blamed on someone else.

Reward determinants

It is now appropriate to look at the specifics of reward management.

The prime determinants of reward, dealt with individually below, are ability to pay, the size or scope of the job to be done, productivity or performance of the workers and competition with other employers for those same workers.

Ability to pay

Most health care organizations, being service organizations, spend some 70% of their annual recurring revenue on wages. The issue is not that the total amount or the proportion is incorrect but that the money is presently not distributed through appropriate mechanisms to the right ends.

On the presumption that no new money is going to be gifted to the organization, then money can be converted by:

- decreasing the number of staff employed;
- lowering the cost of staff by replacing more expensive skills with less expensive;
- restricting overall wage increases to less than the inflation factor in contracts for care; and
- increasing the amount of income-generating work.

Activity

Look at the budget statement for your area of accountability and see how much money you spend on wages and what proportion that is of your total budget.

Divide the number of staff you employ by the budget figure to see the average cost of the labour you employ.

Job size

The Whitley Councils still employ a now out-dated system of job evaluation called 'classification' to place a value on work. This system starts by marking out classes of jobs or occupations and then seeks to describe the broad levels of jobs which may be found in each class. This works so long as managers are only allowed to create jobs which can be found within the classification system and design work accordingly. Classification also only works if the broad levels described actually serve to discriminate between levels in reality i.e. when a hierarchy exists. It quickly becomes apparent that the classification system does not always provide a measure for job size but does dictate:

- the demarcation lines,
- the types of jobs,
- hierarchy, and
- the number of tiers.

Much better job evaluation systems are available to health care organizations than the Whitley Council grading definitions.

The internal structure of remuneration may be based on:

- the responsibility each job has,
- the knowledge and skill the job demands,
- the value to the organization of the output from the job, or
- the amount of resources the job controls.

What is important is that some conscious decision-making takes place about what determines job size so that an appropriate measure can be found.

Once a source of value has been identified and a measure found or invented this must be applied to the jobs required by the organization to do the work effectively. The measure must either just measure without changing the essence of what is being measured or, because a monetary incentive is connected, it must contrive to produce more of what it has been decided is of value. Gender bias is illegal. If the number of staff managed is given a prime place as a factor then people will try to expand their departments and the size of their teams; if budget management is used then budget reductions will be hard to find. Appropriate choices might be knowledge required, problems faced or skills exercised.

When natural clusters of jobs start to emerge from the results then it will all start to look like the contents of a Whitley Council handbook with the difference that it is tailor-made for the organization. Job size measures do not say what pay should be attached to different jobs, they simply rank jobs in size relative to each other. It is an issue worth attention if:

- grade drift is a problem,
- new jobs are needed which Whitley does not classify,
- traditional roles and structures require review, or
- the existing definitions are creating negative behaviour by placing inappropriate values on work.

The last point above is neatly illustrated by highlighting that, while most hospitals are trying to end permanent night working in favour of internal rotation for nurses, a grade 'E' nurse (Whitley grades) is paid the equivalent of a grade 'G' nurse for working those permanent nights or by considering the ancillary off sick on overtime rates referred to above.

Activity

Decide what factor you value most in the task your department performs. Go to the job grading definitions applicable to the staff you manage and see if what you value appears.

Performance

Individual or team performance may matter more than the size of the task to be tackled. Whitley provides little or no scope to reward performance or to create a meritocracy at work. Performance management is covered in Chapter 8. Performance can have a monetary reinforcement but that is not essential or even always desirable. If performance is to be measured and pay is linked to that measure then issues relating to what is valued and who makes the judgments tend to take the focus away from honesty about personal development needs. If lack of competence rather than lack of quantifiable contribution is the problem then a pay link may not be suggested.

People need a certain level of pay to make working an economic proposition. If the money they earn is not considered by them to be as much as they could earn elsewhere they may be demotivated and may depart. Once a wage is achieved which is actually or relatively comfortable a big question exists about whether more money is a motivator toward harder work. Herzberg (1968) separated what he called 'hygiene' factors (like pay, terms and conditions) from 'motivators'. He saw that the work itself and the ability to do a good job and grow professionally were the real motivators to better performance. Pay was important only in that if too low it would cause dissatisfaction.

Vroom (1964) developed a different theory later known as 'expectancy' theory which sees a clear line between what an individual does at work against what that individual expects to obtain. Individuals should, the theory suggests, perceive an available reward, see that reward as attractive and gain it through their efforts. An argument that suggests pay motivates.

Managers do feel that the hard worker who has been in post a year and is 'getting things done' should be paid something more than the long servers who turn up just to 'keep their noses clean'. The 'something more' could be a one-off bonus, a bigger increase or a bigger relative wage.

Introducing performance related pay may:

- increase motivation,
- provide greater equity in reward against effort,
- improve retention of better performers, and
- provide value for something other than long service.

Managers can choose to link reward either to the individual or to the team.

Individual reward

Paying individuals for their own contributions keeps the link between performance and reward very tight and is designed to change work behaviour. Each individual will, it is intended, try to achieve what is valued by the decision-maker. In the health service the system of objective setting for the senior managers worked to ensure that those managers achieved their objectives. If the objectives are not the appropriate ones for success, if other people are upset by instrumental achievement regardless of means or if other priorities arise, then this will matter little to focused achievers. Individual performance related pay provides

reward to individuals for achieving their own objectives even if
their departments collapse.

Team reward

If each individual benefits from the success of their work team
then each member of the team should work for the success of the
whole. Non-achievers will be helped along or pushed out; the
role of the team will be primary and the role of individuals
secondary.

On the other hand, if the team is too large or individuals' roles
are not distinguished, then 'passengers' may develop skills to
hide their lack of contribution behind the success of the others.
Another problem may be that successful individuals just cannot
see their hard work achieving anything in a failing team and so
become demotivated.

Reward can be linked to various measures of performance.
Some examples are:

- output (volume or quality),
- competence,
- achievement of measurable objectives, or
- a share of savings or surplus.

Activity

Which measure of performance is most applicable to your
staff?

Do you know who in your team performs well and if so
consider how you reward them?

Competition

All employees come from the same labour market. They have a
price at which they are prepared to work and health organizations state in their job advertisements the prices they are prepared to pay. Each individual who takes, stays in or leaves a job
has an effect on the overall supply and demand for work and
workers.

If supply and demand are in balance then prices, or in this
case salaries, are likely to hold. If more work exists than people

with the skills to do it then the price will go up. If skills are in over-supply then workers with those skills will drop the price at which they will enter work to ensure that they obtain it, or they will switch to alternative work with a higher rarity value.

The assessing of labour markets is not an exact science. One Trust may find responses to advertisements for support workers number in the hundreds while another Trust in another town nearby cannot recruit. This could be because:

- the labour is not mobile,
- the advertisement was not attractive,
- the advertisement was not displayed in the right place,
- the Trust has a poor reputation as an employer, or
- a competitor is recruiting in the same market.

In this example raising the price would only work in the last instance, and only if the competitor was paying more and pay was clearly the reason for the choices being made. No health organization is a helpless victim of the labour market, but employees and employers are amazingly ignorant about the levels of pay in their local area for different types of work.

Managers should be aware of:

- the state of the local economy,
- the firms operating in their area,
- the skills in demand, and
- local rates of pay.

External rates of pay do represent a reality about the value of work which risks being lost in health care because the health service is an almost monopoly employer of so many skills.

Many skills like those of nurses, doctors, physiotherapists, radiotherapists and medical laboratory officers are all developed for the health service and so a specific organization may gain in the short-term by putting up the price, but unless supply alters recruitment problems will not be solved. If particular managers cannot afford to pay the prices for these skills they should:

- attempt to influence the numbers in training,
- offer less money than the 'going rate' on the basis that supply might exceed overall demand,

- change the methods of work to avoid the need for the expensive skills,
- attempt to obtain the same skills through another route.

Other skills employed in the health service are also utilized by other employers, e.g. porters, personnel managers, plumbers. Demand and supply is not in the control of the health care organization however large an employer it is in the local economy. In these instances the health employer can try to add to its own attractiveness in non-monetary ways in order to recruit and retain the skills needed.

In many cases the Whitley Council rates and conditions far exceed the offer prices needed in the local labour market for transferable skills. There is at present an over-supply of labour and prices for many skills are low. Hospitals are often dramatically over-paying for the labour they employ and could advertise vacancies at considerable reductions. By not doing so they are keeping the prices in the local economy artificially high.

Activity

Make a list of the staff in your team, or the types of staff, and decide for each where their replacement might come from if they were to choose to leave.

Affordability, job size, performance and the 'going rate' all have an impact on pay. Figure 6.1, shows the relationship between different factors which determine reward within a process. The rest of the employment package is made up of terms, conditions and benefits.

Terms and conditions

The relationship between an employee and an employer is regulated by an employment contract. In the health service it is normally written and explicit, giving detail far beyond the 'Statement of particulars' required by law. This contractual document, which includes the relevant Whitley Council handbook or any other documents if referred to, confers rights and liabilities on both parties. For example, it may dictate:

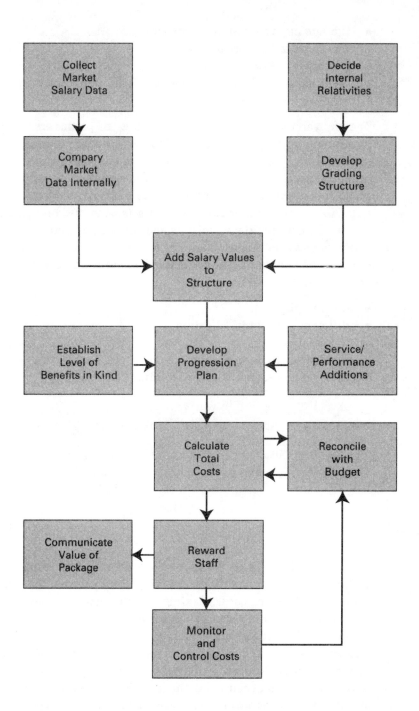

Fig. 6.1 The reward process.

- the rate of pay for Sunday working,
- the hours to be worked in a week,
- guarantees of time off, or
- what happens if the employee is called out for work when off-duty.

Too often all these rules of conduct binding the parties are taken for granted by employer and employees as having to be those enshrined in Whitley – to the inconvenience of both sides. For example, no reasons exist in a Trust for operating department practitioners and nurses, working together in a day surgery unit, to try to function under two different sets of terms concerning hours of work, holidays and unsocial hours payments to the confusion and detriment of all concerned.

Managers should question whether the terms and conditions of their staff are:

- too complicated,
- different without justification,
- too detailed,
- too restrictive on both sides, or
- over generous against what the Trust can afford.

Activity

Given the ability to change your staff's terms and conditions consider which would you choose to alter and why.

Benefits

Many of the benefits or 'perks' of a job are gifted by managers without any right or condition applying. Staff parking, the staff restaurant, discount cards, flexible working hours – these are just some of the many staff privileges and facilities that can be made available. Some can be converted into a monetary value, like lease cars, but most are simply gestures of goodwill. The employees' perceived value of these benefits often exceeds their actual cost. When constructed, the long list of benefits available to staff often makes surprising reading and is worth advertising inside the hospital and out.

Communication

If managers do not reinforce the message then staff will mentally disconnect the wage they receive from the work they do. Employees should understand:

- how much they are paid and for what;
- their grade and how it was determined;
- the method by which their wages increase and the limit to which they can rise;
- any potential for advancement subject to performance and availability of positions; and
- the terms of their employment and the benefits available.

Summary

A real link must be perceived by managers between the amount of the budget spent on wages and the contribution gained from staff.

Pay can be linked to contribution in the following two ways.

- More complex, skilled or responsible work should receive greater reward than less complex or less responsible work so that an incentive exists to acquire skills and responsibility. This requires a mechanism to measure the value of the work people do (job size).

- Secondly, whatever the value of their work, people who work hard and are effective in getting results should be rewarded for their contribution. This requires some form of performance reinforcement for individuals or groups.

If work requires certain specific skills then an eye should be kept to the market place to see what supply and demand do to prices.

This chapter has examined the pay freedoms delegated to health organizations, how those freedoms might be utilized and why.

The prime determinants of reward, taken one at a time, were seen as:

- ability to pay,
- job size,
- performance, and
- competition.

These determinants were seen to relate to each other to produce the reward to staff for work.

Finally terms, conditions, benefits and communication were discussed. The aim has been to create a sense of the real link between the cost of people and their contribution.

Recommended further reading

Managers interested in learning more about this subject should refer to *Reward Management – A Handbook of Salary Administration* by M. Armstrong and H. Murlis, which is published by Kogan Page. Also look at 'Taking Local Management Responsibility for Pay', an article written in 1992 by Peter Haywood and Miranda Vinograd in *Health Manpower Management*, Vol. 18, No. 1. MCB University Press.

References

Department of Health (1989) *Working for Patients: White Paper on the Government's proposals following the review of the NHS.* HMSO, London.

Herzberg, F. (1968) *Work and the Nature of Man.* Staples, London.

Swift, L. (1991) The Pain and Pleasures of Flexible Pay. *Health Manpower Management*, **17**, 11–14.

Vroom, V.H. (1964) *Work and Motivation.* John Wiley & Sons, Chichester.

Further information

Incomes Data Services
193 St John Street
London
EC1V 4LS   0171-250 3434

Chapter 7:
EMPLOYEE RELATIONS

Overview

All too often 'employee relations' is taken to mean relationships between the management and trade unions within a context of collective representation and bargaining. It is important early on to realize that relationships with employees, individually and collectively, and relationships with their representatives are related but different concerns. Managers work with and are part of a team driving toward a common set of work objectives. Managers differ from other members of their teams only in that they hold final authority and responsibility for the task. This role carries with it the responsibility for making decisions that affect the other team members in recruitment, development, retention, promotion, job content, objectives, work levels and processes.

Managers cannot see their team colleagues simply as a resource, like money, buildings or equipment. An economic reality exists in the workplace to demand that managers should see people as such a resource – as a semi-variable cost sunk into the business against which a return is expected. However, this balance sheet does not remove the other reality that people have a whole life outside of work – that they have minds, opinions, emotions, and expectations about life and about work. The need to work with the team while holding managerial authority creates the employee relations agenda.

This agenda is about personal relations, communication, staff grievances, discipline, welfare and dealing with representatives of trade unions or professional associations. Legislation governs the employment relationship in many of the areas listed above.

Many managers think that industrial relations should be the concern of the personnel department and many personnel officers think it the source of their influence. Beaumont (1990) says 'it is likely that the (personnel) function's power will be highly variable through time (e.g. moving up and down as the extent of union power changes)'. Further, he suggests that personnel gain power as a function by adopting procedures to regulate managers' behaviour to meet the needs of employment legislation. Managers, however, should not be leaving the relationship with their staff to a third party.

Learning outcomes

● To see the importance of the individual relationship between managers and each of the employees for whom they are accountable.

● To understand the various organizational means by which the manager/staff relationship is formed and developed.

● To appreciate the type and nature of formal procedures that exist to regulate the behaviour of managers and employees at work.

● To be able to differentiate between formal and informal representation.

● To appreciate that government, through legislation, has a significant role to play in contextualizing workplace employee relations.

Relationships

Managers develop a personal relationship with their own work team whether that relationship is thought about and designed or simply emerges. Any team, large or small, has a view of its manager. This relationship exists between manager and team both at an individual and at a group level. This basic building block is the beginning and end of employee relations.

Any structures or procedures which health organizations put in place to manage employee relations should not serve to distract managers and staff from each other. The wider structures should reinforce, rather than detract from, the primary relationship.

Certain characteristics will exist and have life in managerial and staff relations. Some characteristics may carry values with words like:

- secretive,
- distrustful,
- feared,

- autocratic,
- ruthlessly ambitious.

Others will be positive value characteristics like:

- honest,
- trustworthy,

- respecting,
- fair.

Activity

Think about groups or individuals in your team and write down a few key words you think they might use to describe their relationship with you.

Communication

The life blood of the relationship between managers and their staff is communication. The method of communication, its style, its content, and its delivery all create impressions. Staff need to be able to gain access to their manager to communicate:

- ideas,
- problems and possible solutions,
- concerns and doubts, and
- information on progress.

Equally, the manager needs regular contact with staff to:

- set objectives,
- make observations,
- praise and give feedback,
- advise and inform,
- communicate decisions, and
- consult and involve.

Without this two directional flow work may quickly be disrupted because of:

- lack of information,
- unresolved problems,
- inappropriate action or no action, and
- discontent.

It can be seen from the above that communication is needed to meet certain work-place needs and so is not extra or optional. The need being met or objective sought will dictate the medium, style and content of any organizational communication.

Much communication is found within informal, daily, one-to-one interactions. Managers can promote this important facet of a team's life by giving time to being visible and available in the workplace.

More formal, but still local, communication systems may be necessary for larger groups of health staff.

Workplace meetings

Meetings or briefings are useful to give information to a group, rather than reaching each as an individual, and immediate feedback or reaction is readily obtained. If shift work or internal rotation is a feature then staff may have to stay out of hours or meetings may have to be held more than once. It is also important not to neglect the needs of part-time staff when arranging meetings. However, meetings can be expensive and time consuming.

News sheets and circulars

Written communication which is placed in a reading file, put up on notice-boards or circulated for reading to a named list of individuals is helpful for one-way communication of information. Everyone will see the same thing, but whether messages are really seen, understood or accepted can be difficult to establish.

Activity

List the methods of communication you utilize to communicate with your staff.

Problems with communication systems occur when they:

- do not reach everybody,
- are one-way only,
- do not tell the truth,
- appear to lack managerial commitment,

- omit important information,
- are inconsistent,
- clash with the perceived truth, or
- contain the irrelevant or inconsequential.

A lack of information, attempts to hide or keep back information or a tendency to improve facts in the telling are tactics likely to create cynicism and distrust.

It has been seen then that the relationship between managers and their own staff is at the heart of good employee relations. The life blood of that relationship is sound and direct communication which must be two-way. As this chapter unfolds the primacy of this should not be lost. Managers need to feel confident to deal with their staff before having to resort to formal procedures or set relationships.

Formal procedures

Formal procedures are, according to White (1989), 'procedures which are entered into jointly by management and employee representatives ... designed to ensure that certain standards of industrial behaviour and conduct are adhered to'.

Particular transactions with staff may be accompanied by a need to follow written protocols or procedures to ensure:

- fairness,
- consistency,
- impartiality, and
- a clear route.

Often formal procedures exist concerned with:

- staff grievances,
- incapability,
- ill health or incapacity, and
- misconduct.

Each of these formal areas of employee relations is dealt with below.

Grievances

If a member of staff is disgruntled about some aspect of his or her employment then the manager should be in a position to detect the problem early on. Initial steps should be to:

- give time,
- listen,
- accept the person's feelings, and
- avoid defensive behaviour.

Depending on the problem the manager may then seek to:

- reassure,
- explain,
- provide a fuller perspective,
- provide facts,
- correct any misunderstanding, and
- provide a proposed resolution.

A manager may be unwilling or unable to affect or resolve the perceived problem and so can only explain, clarify and try to provide positive support or some rationale. If the member of staff chooses not to accept the proposed solution or the provided explanation then the grievance remains.

Health organizations typically have a formal grievance procedure available to staff who feel they have a grievance which they have not been able to resolve informally with their manager. In this more formal sense a grievance is a cause for complaint about duties, conditions of service, working conditions or working procedures which may include matters an employee would be entitled to take to an Industrial Tribunal.

Activity

If you do not already know then try and discover whether your organization has a grievance procedure. If it does have one then obtain a copy and familiarize yourself with its contents.

Formal grievance procedures tend to have timescales contained in them to ensure replies to the aggrieved individual from progressive levels of management. The original managers can find themselves, unless careful, polarized in relation to the member of staff – especially if they are required to justify decisions they have made to more senior managers.

This polarization happens usually because the individual employee is not satisfied with the response from the immediate manager. During the operation of the formal grievance procedure and once it is exhausted the manager and the employee must continue to work together. Maintenance of a good relationship is important, even if there has to be an agreement to differ. Neither side should let the situation develop into an 'I win and you lose' scenario. Both sides should recognize the need to make reparation.

Staff can often choose to be represented once a grievance becomes formal and this is discussed later in the chapter.

Case Study – grievance

The role play below, which will take about an hour, highlights a reasonably typical grievance and the different viewpoints of the participants on the same situation.

Employees' brief

You have worked in General Surgery for twenty years. You have been in your current position as Ward Clerk for the last five years and before that you were a Nursing Auxiliary. The change of position related to a back injury sustained when a patient struggled whilst being lifted. As a Ward Clerk you have been working from 9.00 AM to 1.00 PM, Monday through to Friday, which has been ideal as you are able to look after your two grandchildren when they come home from school whilst their mother works part-time on Mondays, Tuesdays and Wednesdays. Your manager has told you that you must now work from 1.00 PM to 5.00 PM, Monday to Friday, as there are too many staff in the mornings and no cover in the afternoons. The other three Ward Clerks in General Surgery are two full-timers and one part-timer. The other part-timer from yourself has been working mornings for six years and has two school age children. Your Statement of Particulars provided five years ago states your hours of work as 20 per week with no times of work specified. You are very upset about the notice of the decision that you should change to afternoon working which appears to you to have been taken without consultation or consideration of your circumstances.

Managers' brief

There has been a recent skill-mix review of the whole of General Surgery as part of a planned revenue savings exercise. Some trained nursing staff have had their jobs placed 'at risk' with the intention that they be replaced by care support workers. It was identified that the number of Ward Clerks in post would remain the same but that better support would be available to other ward staff if there was consistent cover throughout the day shifts. The two full-time ward clerks, who used to work 9.00 AM to 5.00 PM, have agreed to cover early starts and evenings from 7.30 AM to 8.00 PM. The shift payments that would apply increase their earnings. The two part-timers (who currently both work 9.00 AM to 1.00 PM) could between them cover 9.00 AM to 5.00 PM i.e. the 'peak' period. There have been staff briefings about the skill-mix review and the need for change. You were not surprised by the recommendation that the Ward Clerk who has been in post the shortest time should be the one to change her hours. You particularly had the two part-timers contracts drawn up to state the number of hours per week with no specific times to give you the flexibility for just this eventuality.

Staff representative's brief

You are concerned that a number of staff within General Surgery have had to be put up for redeployment because their jobs have been identified as 'at risk' following skill-mix reviews. In regard to the Ward Clerks you do not accept that because the contract only states 20 hours and not specific times the manager can unilaterally change the times worked. You consider this a fundamental breach of contract and that the member of staff has the 'right' to work 9.00 AM to 1.00 PM through accepted and established practice.

The agreed outcome that you arrive at in this case study is not important as long as agreement can be reached by all the participants.

Incapability

Expectation about the capabilities of employees should take into account:

- skills and qualifications held,
- volume of work to be done,
- procedures or processes to be followed, and
- standards of quality expected.

If standards exist then managers should make them explicit in:

- recruitment literature,
- job descriptions,
- personnel specifications,
- objectives, and
- work procedures or manuals.

Recruitment

Careful screening at the stage of recruitment and selection of employees can mean the long and painful process of dealing with employees who cannot do their job is avoided.

Obvious examples exist where unsuitable candidates can be excluded through proper recruitment screening. Jobs involving driving can have a selection criterion which demands the holding of a full driving licence with no penalties or endorsements. The manager can then be reasonably sure that the new employee is capable of driving and driving to an acceptable standard, although this should be followed up at interview by questions on the amount and nature of driving practice.

Where skills are less easily transparent, like clerical checking, then a test or work sample exercise could be considered or proof of previous work performed to a sufficient standard might be sought.

It may be unfair for a manager to have known that certain skills and experience were required in a job, to have failed to test for those skills and still to have recruited a candidate 'as seen' only to later accuse the member of staff of incapability.

Induction

The standard of work required should be explained to new employees during their induction programme so that they are left in no doubt as to the standards expected of them and what support they can expect. In addition the consequences of any failure to meet the required standards should be explained. Having such information is essential to the new employee to ensure their success in their new role.

Process

Employees are recruited on a judgment, tested or not, that they can do the job. If a manager becomes concerned that a new or previously satisfactory employee is not performing then something has gone wrong. In these circumstances managers should:

- draw the problem to the employee's attention,
- seek an explanation,
- make clear the standards expected,
- provide training and support to remedy any deficiency in knowledge or skill,
- caution the employee about the consequences of failure to meet the required standards,
- give the employee the opportunity to improve; and
- monitor progress to provide feedback.

Activity

Select a job in your structure that you know reasonably well and think about what is expected from its holder.

Ask yourself about the standards you have or the expectations you place on the postholder.

Are those standards made explicit, are they known by and made available to the postholder?

Did the original recruitment exercise seek to predict the employee's success at meeting the standards expected?

Formal action

Procedures for dealing with incapability tend to suggest that the manager who alleges it demonstrates the basis of this belief to a more senior manager. That more senior manager will want to see evidence of poor performance but also that the above processes have been followed. In most instances the employee will receive a first warning and then later a final one if work does not improve.

Remedies can include:

- further training,
- a period of supervision or mentoring,
- relocation to other equivalent duties,
- demotion to less demanding work, or
- dismissal.

Ill-health or incapacity

Ill-health is another but more specific form of incapability. The health service more than any other employer should respect that not everyone enjoys good health all the time. Indeed, hospitals, surgeries and health clinics are a collection point and breeding ground for causes of poor health. Employees, depending on their employment terms and length of service, have an entitlement to paid sickness absence which, from time to time, they may need.

The above, while true, does not mean that managers should ignore staff absence. Absence patterns in different parts of the service and in different occupations are predictable across groups of staff. Particular individuals or groups may either have good or bad attendance levels against what is acceptable or accepted as normal. A high level of absence may arise from a particular spell of long absence or else repeated short-term absences.

Long-term absence

The important factors in long term absence are the contractual paid entitlement to absence, the predicted length of time to full recovery and return to work, and how long the workplace can manage without the employee. If an employee is going to make a full recovery within the entitlement to absence, then it is best to give support in that recovery and return.

If the employee is not likely to make a sufficient recovery, or not within the entitlement to absence or pay, then that fact is best faced by both the employee and the manager as soon as it is clear. No good comes from continuing the employment relationship against the face of the medical facts.

Persistent short-term absence

It is important in cases of short-term absence to look for an underlying medical reason that may link the absences and indicate them to be because of a particular cause of poor health. If no medical or other related reason links or explains the absences then misconduct might be indicated.

Presuming that medical reasons exist for each absence, or for the repeated absences, then the length of time required to make a full recovery should be considered against the entitlement to absence and the effect of the absences on the workplace. An employee with health that is generally poor, but without a single underlying cause that can be identified and treated, does not have to be retained. As with other categories of incapability, a period of probation is normally allowed to give the employee an opportunity to improve.

In all ill-health absence cases medical advice and reports should be obtained from the occupational health physician if one exists or from the employee's general practitioner.

Remedies can include:

- advice to seek treatment,
- time to recover,
- redeployment to other equivalent duties,
- redeployment to lighter duties or fewer hours of work, or
- dismissal.

In deciding the appropriate action where there is no likelihood of an improvement in attendance, the length of service and absence record of the employee should be considered alongside the availability of alternative work and the effect of the absences within the workplace. Pregnancy is not ill-health and inability to undertake work due to pregnancy should be dealt with by suspension on full pay or redeployment rather than dismissal, which is prohibited by statute. This would be the case, for example, with some jobs in departments such as X-ray, theatre, portering, radiotherapy or isotope imaging.

Case Study – ill-health

The following role play, which will take about half an hour, will create a sense of some of the tensions and emotions that tend to lie behind meetings concerning an individual employee's attendance record.

Employee's brief

You are a staff nurse on a medical ward and have worked for the last three years on the same ward. In the winter just gone the ward on which you work had an outbreak of diarrhoea and vomiting which affected both staff and patients. That outbreak along with the normal winter colds that went around meant you had three short absences from work. In the spring your two children seemed to pick up colds from school and inevitably they brought their infections into the home and again you had a period of absence. You thought it better to stay at home when you had an infection rather than bring it into the ward environment with the associated risks. You were recently sent by your manager to see the hospital's Occupational Health Physician and it was no surprise to you, having subsequently received a copy of the medical report, that there was no underlying health problem linked with your recent absences from work. You have now been asked to visit your manager in the office at a pre-arranged time. You are not concerned about this appointment as you were genuinely ill on each occasion of your absence and you are fit and healthy. You are not, as you perceive it, one of those people who just takes the odd day off on sick leave for the slightest of reasons.

Manager's brief

You are a manager of four medical wards. You have been sent a copy of a recent district audit report which criticized the department you manage for its high level of short-term absenteeism and suggested a more positive management approach. The cost of absence for each speciality has been highlighted and you have had to cover sickness absence with bank or agency nurses which created an adverse budget position. To respond you have pulled out of your attendance records all those staff with more that 20 days' absence in the last year and have arranged Occupational Health appointments for those people. You have been advised that if no underlying health problem exists to link episodes of short-term absence then the matter can be dealt with as a disciplinary issue depending on individual circumstances. You are now seeing those individuals whose Occupational Health medical reports indicates that they do not have an underlying health problem causing their absences from work. The objective is to counsel them and to decide whether or not to proceed with more formal action. Your next appointment is to see one of the staff nurses.

Misconduct

The organization will have rules of conduct and expectations about behaviour. In the same way each manager will have to think about their own rules and expectations so as to make them explicit and specific to their own work situation.

Obvious rules will exist surrounding:

- theft,
- assault,
- fraud,
- confidentiality,
- negligence, and
- insubordination.

Other areas such as appearance, hours of work, standards of conduct and compliance with safety procedures may need to be tailored to the particular workplace.

Each offence should have a clear penalty, where penalties are appropriate, so that employees know which sanction is appropriate. For example, theft will produce dismissal regardless of the circumstances whereas poor time-keeping may result in an informal review or perhaps a first warning depending on the reason and the degree. Real life throws up problems that are less than clear, such as suspected theft through fraudulent travel claims or verbal rather than physical assault and so managers must make their own judgments.

Disciplinary procedures tend to give different levels of managers the ability to take disciplinary action up to and including dismissal. Such procedures also give a structure to disciplinary hearings so that they are conducted fairly. Minimum requirements are that the employee:

- hears the allegation made and the nature of any evidence to substantiate it,
- has an opportunity to reply or explain,
- can call witnesses and produce statements,
- can be represented, and
- can appeal.

Disciplinary action may include:

- taking no formal action,
- written warnings,
- action short of dismissal, e.g. disciplinary down-grading,
- dismissal with notice,
- summary dismissal.

Warnings issued should be in force for a specified time with further misconduct leading to further more severe sanctions.

Safety

Managers have a duty to their staff in connection with health and safety at work; they must provide a safe place of work. This is the minimum legal requirement. Beyond this minimum managers should be concerned with the work environment, the conditions in which staff have to work and observance of the regulations which are many and complex. Care and attention should be given to the place of work to provide a situation in which people can productively spend a large proportion of their time. If safety legislation (e.g. The Health and Safety at Work Act 1974) is not complied with and the lack of compliance is due to a manager's neglect then the individual can be found guilty as well as the employing organization.

In large organizations, like health services, managers tend to accept the condition of staff residences, ward areas, receptions and clinic rooms as given. The works, estates or capital planning department is mentally allocated responsibility for the infrastructure and work surroundings. Occupational health, personnel or safety teams are allocated the role of ensuring safe workplaces. It is true that if such departments do exist then they have some contribution but that is not to distract managers from their primary responsibility. Peeling walls and crowded offices communicate to employees. The work environment may include such things as:

- decor,
- heating,
- lighting,
- location,
- space,
- equipment, and
- substances.

Each department should have developed a written statement of its health and safety policy rules or regulations specific to that department's workplace and its specific risks. Ideally, the document should be signed and dated by the manager as its 'owner'. The statement should seek to identify individuals with special roles in the department and their responsibilities, e.g. safety representative, first aider, safety auditor and so on.

The manager should be familiar with certain key local procedures such as those contained in with the Control of Substances Hazardous to Health Regulations 1988, the Reporting of Injuries, Disease and Dangerous Occurrences Regulations 1985, the Electricity at Work Regulations 1989 and such European Community Directives as affect health services e.g. manual handling, visual display units etc.

To make any policy or regulations meaningful to a specific workplace the manager should identify potential causes of accidents and assess the risk of those hazards. Consulting previous accident records may be helpful in that regard.

Counselling

Managers often find themselves as the first point of contact for employees to discuss their problems, generated both inside and outside work. This seems to be because managers:

- are available,
- are in perceived positions of authority,
- are often respected,
- can allow time off, and
- can make allowances for problems at work if aware of their causes.

It is important that managers take their role as a listening ear seriously. Occasionally, some encouragement to seek further expert advice is appropriate.

Informal representation

Individual

Some employees do not feel confident in one to one situations when they feel they have something difficult or significant to say or find themselves involved in any of the above procedures. In some cases they may ask for a friend or work colleague to be present to support them or to speak on their behalf. By allowing individuals to do this and acting sensitively managers will build the relationship so that in future the employees may feel more confident to speak for themselves.

Group

A work group may feel it has a collective or shared view about a work related issue and the members of that group may want to express the commonly held view to their manager, either as individuals or as a group. Groups normally then either elect someone to speak on their behalf or write a joint letter which each individual signs. Again, a positive acknowledgement and response to the whole group, or to each individual member, will tend to diffuse any difficult situation.

Formal representation

A proportion of the staff in the health service have chosen to join a trade union or professional association, usually for individual protection of their rights. Because staff have chosen to join these trade or professional organizations, the officials of that organization may attempt to claim a share in the manager's power to make decisions. Managers need to consider their options carefully and decide on a strategy. With the existence of Trusts and the long predicted demise of the national Whitley Councils the focus is shifting from the national scene to local health managers. Trade unions are rightly concerned about the new freedoms of these managers to make decisions which affect their members.

In formal procedures such as grievance or discipline the involved staff, if they are trade union members, will often choose to exercise their right to be represented.

Some managers believe they can negate the need for their staff to join unions, that employee rights do not need defending in fear in their department, hospital or locality. In such instances, staff joining trade unions and bringing in representatives may be seen as an insult to the manager's integrity. Other managers would encourage their staff to join trade unions and prefer to deal through representatives rather than with the staff directly.

The wider organization may have made its own decision about whether or not to recognize all or some trade unions for wider collective consultation or bargaining purposes. 'Collective bargaining' is the term used where recognized representatives of a collective group negotiate in a way which then excludes any opportunity for individuals to agree through their own separate exchange (Potter, 1891).

Thirty-four trade unions claim recognition at the national level. Local health organizations, if they have chosen to recognize trade unions, may have:

- recognized all trade unions who have any members among the staff,
- recognized those trade unions with a significant membership base within the staff group they purport to represent, or
- recognized one trade union for each major staff group.

Alternatively, a decision may have been taken to resist any form of recognition having instead:

- management communication,
- elected employee councils (works councils), and
- other forms of employee participation.

Personnel directors will put in place local machinery for pay determination which may bring with it trade union recognition.

This may have some effect on managers' own reactions as individuals to the explicit presence in their departments of active union members seeking consultation or negotiation.

Managers need to consider:

- how many staff are members of unions,
- which unions have members, and
- whether there are any representatives or stewards.

Managers can choose to:

- deal with representatives solely for individual representation of specific members,
- keep representatives informed of management issues,
- consult with representatives before decisions are made, and
- negotiate with representatives on specific issues, making decisions by agreement.

Representatives of employees may seek to expand the coverage and the depth of detail of managers' discussions with them. If they are powerful enough they will increase their expectations about being consulted or negotiated with and seek settlements or concessions which are beneficial to them. Managers need to be aware of staff-side representatives' perceptions of their relative power to affect decision-making. Managers often need to co-operate with representatives at least to the extent of preserving their relationship. Local representatives may involve full-time officers to support them on particular issues. It may be that full-time officers are allowed to attend and make representations only by agreement or until the local representatives become more confident.

The health service may be in a transitional stage toward a post-bargaining era where some other local mechanism will exist to settle staff terms. These new arrangements may be based on systematic and technical data such as job evaluation results, market surveys and affordability rather than on the relative bargaining power of the parties. In that light, perhaps each Trust should have a single independent but expert review body which would make recommendations to the Trust Board.

Legislation

Political background

In the early 1960s no employment legislation existed of any merit. Developments in employment law since that time have fallen into two parts, those statutes introduced prior to 1979 and those introduced since. The major employment relations laws introduced before 1979 include:

- The Redundancy Payments Act 1965,
- The Equal Pay Act 1970,
- The Industrial Relations Act 1971,
- The Employment of Children Act 1973,
- The Trade Union and Labour Relations Act 1974,
- The Health and Safety at Work Act 1974,
- The Employment Protection Act 1975,
- The Sex Discrimination Act 1975,
- The Race Relations Act 1976, and
- The Employment Protection (Consolidation) Act 1978.

The titles comprising this tide of statutes give away their intentions. Trade unions and individual rights in employment developed in this period within an increasingly restrictive employment framework. The coverage of these Acts included:

- trade union recognition and closed shop agreements;
- trade union membership rights;
- the outlawing of sex and race discrimination in employment;
- bargaining and collective agreements, including compulsory disclosure of information to trade unions;
- industrial action and immunity from legal action;
- the concept of unfair dismissal, including placing the onus of proof on to the employer; and
- extended individual employment rights.

The Conservative Government which came into power in 1979 also saw employment issues as a political priority and passed the following major legislation:

- The Employment Act 1980,
- The Employment Act 1982,
- The Trade Union Act 1984,
- The Employment Act 1988,
- The Employment Act 1989,
- The Employment Act 1990,
- The Trade Union and Labour Relations (Consolidation) Act 1992,
- The Trade Union Reform and Employment Rights Act 1993.

The titles of the Acts in this second wave of legislation are not as imaginative and they do not provide the same clues as to content (making the life of any personnel management student more difficult). However, much of the content of the above Acts was addressed to releasing the employment market from the first list above. The themes included:

- providing for democracy within trade unions, including rules about ballots and election of officials;
- restricting industrial action rights, including picketing and secondary action;
- restricting trade unions' immunity from legal action by employers and others;
- restricting the trade unions' expenditure for explicitly political purposes;
- reducing employee rights by increased qualifying periods of employment for unfair dismissal claims; and
- giving rights to trade union members against their trade union, including removal of support for closed shops.

European influence

Much of the legislation introduced to further increase the rights of employees at work has been driven by the European Community. The perception is, however, that the influence of European labour policy on the UK has been accepted only reluctantly. For example, the Equal Pay Act 1970, passed five years prior to its enforcement date, did not meet the requirements of the European Equal Pay Directive adopted by member states in 1975. It took the government two attempts to bring the domestic legislation into line, the Equal Pay (Amendment)

Regulations 1983 and the Sex Discrimination and Equal Pay (Remedies) Act 1993.

This amount of law and its complexity, if not contradiction, at national and European levels, can catch managers on the wrong side of the line in their own practices. Two cases in 1993 demonstrated this difficulty: *Marshall* v. *Southampton and South West Hampshire Area Health Authority* and *Enderby* v. *Frenchay Health Authority and the Secretary of State for Health.* Both these cases fell through the gap between domestic and European legislation on equality. British governments have a consistent record of failing fully to implement European legislation and managers are often the victims.

Managers should attempt to keep up to date with or obtain advice on employment legislation and ensure that the procedures that they operate adhere to the requirements of law.

Activity

Obtain a copy of the Trade Union and Employment Rights Act 1993, or a summary of it, from your library or personnel department. You will find within this Act that employees are to receive a written statement of the terms of their employment called a principal statement. Make a list of what should be included in this statement and compare it with your own statement of employment particulars.

Summary

The relationship of managers with their own staff is the foundation of the employment relationship. Managers relate to individuals and to groups in the workplace. Those groups or individuals may choose to be represented in formal proceedings or may wish to be consulted. The need for good practice and to meet legislative requirements can mean managers having to follow written procedures in certain situations like staff misconduct. Many of the formal arrangements between employee and employer are governed by legislation.

Recommended further reading

Recognising Trade Unions by Nancy Harding and Peter Haywood, 1991, published by North West Thames Regional Health Authority Pay Unit, in their PAYFOLIO series, provides a useful analysis of matters covered in this chapter.

References

Beaumont, P.B. (1990) *Change in Industrial Relations*. Routledge, London.

Potter, B. (1891) *The Co-operative Movements in Great Britain*. Allen and Unwin, London.

White, P.J. (1989) Industrial Relations Procedures. In *A Handbook of Industrial Relations Practice* (ed. B. Towers). Kogan Page, London.

Further Information

Advisory, Conciliation & Arbitration Service
Head Office
27 Wilton Street
London
SW1X 7AZ   0171 210 3000

Chapter 8:
PERFORMANCE

Overview

It is important for managers to both get the best out of people and enable them to give of their best. Performance management is therefore one of the key roles of any manager. In the same way the finance director looks for the maximum return on capital employed so managers, assisted by human resource professionals, will want to maximize return from the human asset, but without causing over heating.

Health professionals, and other employees, will want to use to the full the skills they have gained and, on the whole, will want to find a challenge in their work. They will want to gain a sense of achievement from their work and to ensure directly or indirectly that the best care for patients is provided. Managers and staff in this sense have a single shared objective.

It is therefore in the interests of both management and staff to have in place systems and processes which ensure that staff can give a full contribution to care and that the employer gets a return on its investment. To achieve the above, organizations or departments need to design plans to develop the potential of staff and improve job performance by providing clear objectives so that individual employee efforts assist the total Trust in its objective of providing health care.

This chapter will examine what is meant by performance in a care environment and how it can be measured. It will look at performance management plans, and different performance environments. Finally it explores concerns about what is input to a work system to gain a performance outcome and how those outcomes might be assessed.

Learning outcomes

- To appreciate the nature of performance as it can be understood and measured in a health care context.

- To understand the concept of 'customers' in health care

and the different customers that exist depending on the specific service being considered.

● To gain familiarity with performance management processes and the need to design a performance management plan.

● To appreciate the role of reviewing historical performance against chosen criteria, including appraisal for individuals.

● To have considered the importance, or otherwise, of monetary reward in sustaining high performance.

What is performance?

A common dictionary definition is 'a carrying out of something: something done'. What that 'something' may be is left to the subjective and often fertile imagination. The important thing about this definition is that it is something 'done'. Much of what occurs in health care looks like a set of processes and behaviours that have no discernible outcome. This is part of the service's complexity rather than its measurement difficulty. Care staff find it difficult to imagine that what they do can be quantified. How can care be measured? The answer is that in the purest sense care cannot be measured. However, within a Trust care has a purpose and an outcome and therefore the component parts of care can be measured. It is possible to measure:

● productivity (more from less),
● effectiveness (more of the right thing),
● efficiency (smarter working), and
● quality (getting it right).

Performance units

These measures refer not only to front-line clinical services but also to intermediate services back from the front line. The health service is large and complex and that complexity cannot be ignored when examining performance. Health organizations are made up of different services described below.

Primary providers

Surgery, Medicine, Learning Disabilities, and so on, provide direct care and support to patients and clients and so are examples of primary providers. It is these services which typically seek health care contracts from purchasers so gaining income for the Trust.

Secondary providers

Theatres, out-patients, X-ray, convalescent homes, and so on, while providing services to patients or clients, do so in support of the primary service and so are secondary providers. The primary providers have to include, or absorb in their plans for work, the cost and capacity of these secondary services.

Providers within providers

A whole series of services exist which lie behind the primary and secondary providers and which are essential to their operation. These provide their services to the primary and secondary providers internally. The purpose of these organizations is not patient care. Pharmacy, portering, catering, haematology, and so on, all fall into this category. The important thing about these services is that their workload has a direct relationship to the changing workload of the primary and secondary care providers.

Overheads

A series of services then exist which provide a framework for the whole; these have a stable cost structure, and are relatively insensitive to changing patient workload. These services generate no income but form a necessary shared overhead on the business, e.g. management, finance, personnel.

The 'something done' covered by each of these different classifications of the whole will be different. The people employed will have different outputs in mind in doing their jobs and will be working for different customers. These different components of the health service form a chain, each linking to the other.

> ## Activity
>
> Decide where the service you manage falls in the above process chain.
>
> List the customers of your service, whether they be general practitioners, purchasing authorities, or other service departments.

The importance of customers

Rather than each service in the above chain reaching its own conclusions about the outputs it is to deliver, this information should be obtained from the customers, internal or external, with which it has links. Recognizing the customer and establishing their requirements gives the most appropriate performance definition available to service organizations like health services. Customer requirements often exceed or take for granted requirements found in the best self-generated professional specifications. A long list of customers may exist around the hospital or community. The process of defining their requirements may involve a prolonged episode of introductions, establishing relationships and information gathering.

The object of such an exercise must be to gain a clear view of the important outputs and the criteria by which those outputs are to be measured. As Brinkerhoff and Dressler (1990) say, 'Customer expectations, needs, and opinions for quality form the basis for specifying measurable quality criteria that will be incorporated into the output component of the productivity ratio'. For front-line services quantity, cost, quality, waiting time and information requirements will feature in the mix. For intermediate services the issues include responsiveness, flexibility and cost. These measures are the definition of performance for the organization and the individuals in it. The challenge is to relate customer requirements back to the individual employee's contribution.

While a retail shop assistant's service at the checkout till may assist the business by bringing the customer back to the shop, a quality service provided by an outpatient reception clerk may not produce the same link with customer loyalty. However, if the patient came from a general practitioner fundholder and the clerk failed accurately to collect the appropriate information to allow an invoice to be raised the Trust's finances and reputation would suffer.

Measurement

Having found the critical performance indicators the next step towards using the human resource more efficiently is the ability to measure the current level of performance. Such measures will, by necessity, be relative in that they will only be useful when comparisons are made with other similar units at the same time. Variations in performance within one unit or between units directs the manager's attention to reasons for the variations and so to improvements in the less well performing units. Staff are an expensive input to the health care system and so any measure should examine that input and the relationship between it and the outcome sought. Possible measures for human resources are:

- average staff costs,
- output per member of staff,
- output per pound spent on wages, or
- staff costs as a proportion of total costs.

The output measures in the above ratios would depend on the service and what its customers perceive as important from it, which could be:

- out-patients seen,
- in-patients discharged,
- items of laundry cleaned,
- theatre packs made up, or
- test results provided.

The ratios can work to measure the performance of individuals, teams and departments over time. More importantly those individuals, teams or departments can be compared with each other and the contribution each makes recognized.

To use such measures the information has to be available and reliable over a period of time. Those subject to the measure and those receiving the information generated have to see it as relevant. More importantly, for human measures the staff used as the input side of the ratio have to be able to affect the output side in their daily work.

Performance management plans

Knowing what to measure and how to measure it does not in isolation make for good performance management. The management of performance is far wider than the conduct of reviews of performance. A plan to improve performance in an organization should seek to integrate:

- departmental objectives,
- wider organizational demands,
- role descriptions and targets,
- performance monitoring,
- performance reviews,
- reward for success,
- identification of training needs, and
- management of poor performance.

Figure 8.1 shows a possible performance management process linking the above factors. Performance management is, therefore, a total management concept and culture. It flows through every aspect of the operation. All managers must ask the following questions:

- What is the Trust business plan?
- What have I to achieve to meet the plan?
- How do I best achieve the plan?
- How do I monitor progress?
- How do I reward those who contribute?

Environment

It is the people who convert hospital buildings, beds, pharmaceutical products and theatre packs into environments for caring and curing. It is the people who turn pool cars and dressing packs into community care. The health organization only performs if its people perform. What distinguishes care from treatment is the way in which people go about their jobs. Performance needs to be considered in terms of behaviour as well as outcomes. Creating the right environment for better performance is critical to performance improvement.

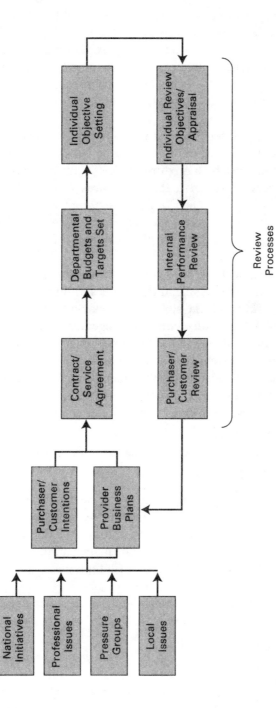

Fig. 8.1 An example of a performance management process.

Alternative styles

The nature of the performance plan introduced will depend on the individual manager's style and orientation. Douglas McGregor (1960) described two contrasting assumptions about the behaviour of employees which he called 'theory X' and 'theory Y'.

Broadly, theory X took the view that the average employee disliked work, tried to avoid responsibility and could only be made to work by a mixture of close control and threat.

Theory Y assumed that work was a natural and welcome activity which need not be externally controlled as the employee was already adequately motivated. Employees would seek responsibility and give valuable help in solving work problems.

McGregor took the view that theory Y was the correct assumption to make and that firms should be organized on that basis. Theory X is similar to task-centred management and theory Y to people-centred management. McGregor felt that a large fund of valuable expertise, experience and originality among employees was often untapped by management.

Theory Y postulated that management strategy should be aimed at creating conditions which enabled each individual to achieve personal goals by directing their efforts towards organizational goals.

Management by objectives

McGregor saw 'Management by objectives' as an application of his theory Y. Management by objectives is a method of defining the role of subordinates and setting specific targets for them within set time limits. The manager then supports and encourages the subordinates so that they can reach the set objectives.

The phases to be considered in developing performance management plans are:

● the organizational,
● the mechanistic, and
● the human.

Activity

Do the staff you manage have written job descriptions?

Obtain a copy of one of the job descriptions, if they exist, and ask whether it simply describes tasks to be done or whether it lays stress on that post's unique responsibility.

Phase 1: organizational

The part of the organization for which any manager is responsible is one part of a wider system. Each part has inputs and outputs just as the whole organization has inputs and outputs. The fact that the organization seems to be designed as it is found does not make that design the most efficient or effective. Managers should ask whether the particular cell they manage and its sub-parts:

● are structurally well placed,
● are geographically well placed,
● enter the work process at the right time,
● should exist in their current form, or
● should exist at all.

Case study – sources of personnel services

A central department of personnel specialists exists as a funded team to support various managers in decision-making about staff management. It has been asked in an organizational context whether the team should:

● continue to exist as a funded central team,

● have its services tendered competitively,

● enter into service agreements with users,

● devolve its budgets and trade with users,

● devolve all its resources including staff to users, or

● cease to exist and release the resources for another purpose.

As a manager to whom this service is provided which option would you prefer?

By more appropriately designing the organization and its work processes at the macro level greater leaps in performance gain may be possible.

Another aspect of the organizational model is related to the inside of each organizational cell. Some organizations should appropriately have a technical hierarchy, others are better able to achieve through teams of equals or temporary groupings of people with the skills to tackle particular tasks. The traditional bureaucracies found within health services are rarely the best way to organize labour in service organizations, but are better suited to control cultures.

This organizational aspect was explored in Chapter 5 on Labour utilization.

Phase 2: mechanistic

Each post, in this second stage, will have a clear job description setting out outcomes expected which link back to the key purpose of that job in the organization. The sum of the outcomes of each individual job description will add up to the task expected from the organization. All postholders will know from their job descriptions why their particular job exists and how it contributes to the overall purpose.

As each job has a clear and distinct purpose then the accountability which rests with each is clear. Posts which rely on others to deliver goods or services need to have those others accountable to them so that the chain of responsibility matches the flow of work. Such lines of accountability can be drawn diagrammatically. The organizational structure chart which evolves from this process can be shared with each participant.

Relatively timeless statements of accountability in job descriptions can be broken down on a regular basis into current steps or objectives for each employee in the structure. The progress of the organization and of individuals can then be monitored through management by objectives and problem identification.

Phase 3: human

Managers should audit the skills at their disposal in the team which is to carry out the task. This skills audit can be compared with an assessment of the skills required. Improved performance is gained here by placing individuals in the jobs which are designed to demand their skills profile. In this way people have their roles shaped around them to play to their strengths and so can maximize the contribution they can make. Skills deficiencies identified in the team as a whole (and in particular individuals) can become the subject of organizational and individual development plans.

Promoting individual and team development in this way gains the commitment of the team who then tend to behave in a motivated and directed way. All individuals are developed to their maximum potential so that their contribution to the organization is maximized.

In such a skills based model managers, by encouraging appropriate behaviours, can act as role models or 'learning leaders' rather than 'controllers'.

Activity

Do the staff you manage have personal development plans?

Do those plans allow you to compare individuals skills and behaviours against their job requirements?

The three approaches described above are not mutually exclusive and each could play a part in the overall plan developed to manage performance.

Role profiles

Individual employees, in the 'mechanistic' phase described above, are said to require job descriptions which set out the unique contribution of each person's role. Such descriptions can serve a wide range of purposes. As well as the employees understanding their own personal contribution they can, through role profiles, understand the roles of other associated individuals and how they inter-relate with their respective contributions in a team. By understanding their role boundaries individuals can be empowered to act within their field of responsibility. In the 'human' phase described above, it would be appropriate to include in the role profile the acceptable competence level required for the job. Increasingly, this competence framework is being provided through National Vocational Qualifications. Job analysis is a useful tool and was described in more detail in Chapter 5.

Performance reviews

Having appropriate measures (and a plan to enable improvement) it is now possible to look at review systems. A well defined appraisal system is essential for any manager wishing to manage performance. Managers should not feel bound to follow a set administrative procedure for conducting performance review or appraisal if the provided system is irrelevant to their work team or environment, but it is important that the goals are common. If reward is attached then the measurement outcome may have to be common amongst managers. Performance review can be a review of:

- departments,
- teams,
- individuals, or
- all the above in sequence.

Choices exist to review:

- outputs,
- targets or ratios,
- objectives,
- observed behaviours, and
- proven competence or skills.

The appraisal system can be based on:

- management appraisal of subordinates,
- peer appraisal of each other,
- upward appraisal,
- self-appraisal, or
- customer appraisal of the team.

To appraise requires planning in advance to set goals or desired outcomes, driven from customer need, against historical performance. A review can then compare the new situation with that which went before and the new situation against the target sought.

Appraisal

Appraisal interviews are often viewed by the assessor and the assessed as difficult. Perhaps this perception exists because so much weight was placed on a traditionally held annual event which for senior managers and senior nurses in the health service had also been the focus of discussion about their annual pay award. Appraisal need be neither difficult nor linked to pay.

The normal rules which govern good interviewing govern appraisal. The assessor should:

- prepare,
- give advance notice,
- set aside adequate time,
- avoid interruptions,
- avoid any surprises,
- be objective and factual,
- ask open-ended questions, and
- let the interviewee do the talking.

If specific advice exists for appraisal then it is to:

- praise positively,
- criticize constructively,
- keep a balance,
- place the emphasis on future performance, and
- consider development needs.

Rewards for success

In the sense that employees should be the subject of formal proceedings which may lead to their dismissal if they do not deliver a satisfactory performance then the whole of any employee's pay is performance related. This at least sets a minimum standard of performance.

Whether to reward

Beyond this point disagreement exists between managers, with three typical points of view:

- that motivation is intrinsic,
- that money motivates, or
- that gains should be shared fairly.

Motivation is intrinsic

Some believe that staff are either motivated or they are not and that appealing to an employee's need for material gain will not make any difference to their inherent motivation level. Monetary inducement will simply cause instrumental behaviour designed to get the reward. In health services a strong argument exists that staff are motivated to deliver the standards of care they have been trained to provide. As Handy (1994) puts it 'the wealth creation of a business is as worth doing and as valuable as the health creation of a hospital'.

Money motivates

Others think that pay plays a large part in the employee's reason for being at work and that performance will improve if a monetary reward lies at the end. A point exists to working harder if individual employees know they will gain cash or other benefits.

Just share of gains

Other managers believe that it is only right that if performance or productivity improves which releases money, then employees should get a fair share for their part in that achievement.

Types of reward

On being able to distinguish that one team or individual is doing better than another places with some managers the wish to reward the better team or individual. The rewards the manager may have in mind include:

- recognition or praise,
- future stability,
- investment in staff or equipment, and
- better training or promotion prospects.

All of these benefits are within the manager's scope and are often influenced by feedback to the manager about performance levels. Other areas of reward for better performing teams or individuals are more controversial:

- the one-off non-recurring bonus (gain share or award schemes),

- increases to basic pay,
- prizes (e.g. dinner-for-two vouchers).

Points of controversy

Problems of fairness and equity of treatment make the application of money for performance gain controversial.

What to measure?

The first problem is the measure. Is the manager going to measure and judge success by:

- the effort put in,
- the results achieved, or
- the effect of those results?

Case study – measuring for reward

Two ward teams are allocated projects at the beginning of the year. One group of staff worked all hours against the odds to produce a hard earned result which although important was not critical to success. The neighbouring team had a high profile project which they enjoyed delivering and it had a significant impact on the organization's success. The reward of effort in, results out, or contribution made are important questions. Which determinant do you choose in this example?

Affordability

The second problem is one of affordability in the public services. Some departments may be involved in trading accounts and activities which bring in both internal and external revenue, typically the pharmacy, the laundry or the works department. If they do more work, raise their prices or find efficiency savings then additional revenue is earned, some of which could be made available to the employees. Other departments, typically X-ray, pathology and finance, have no means of raising income as they operate from delegated budgets providing a free service at source. Also, while raising prices in the trading departments generates more income, the employees are doing nothing extra to be entitled to claim a share of the increased profit.

Proper use of public money

As health service money is mainly public money and efficiency is expected of public services, why should the remedy for past inefficiency mean money being paid into the pockets of today's individuals? If clinical services can deliver patient care at the volumes set in contracts, at less than the contract price, are they not robbing other patients of care by charging higher prices? Savings should perhaps be recycled internally or through purchasers to increase the amount of patient care that can be delivered in the future. This thinking negates any legitimacy in productivity bonuses, but it is an issue to be considered.

Training needs

Identifying the changing needs of the organization and providing the skills to meet those needs is an important product of performance management. Employees will join the organization, change jobs and will leave so changing the stock of skills available to any manager. At the same time the task and its demands will change. Identifying the need for skills and ensuring the provision of those skills in new or existing staff will ensure continued ability to meet the demands of the task. This will require an analysis of:

- the task to be done,
- the skills necessary for the task,
- the skills available, and so
- the skills gap.

The overall review process

It is necessary to discover at the end whether:

- the organization is actually performing any better than it was;
- the performance management system being used remains appropriate;
- the human resources employed contributed to any improved performance.

Managers should ensure a process exists within teams and departments to conduct major service reviews utilizing:

- data from information systems such as staff numbers, activity, budgets and quality;
- reports from scrutiny systems such as ward audit, control of infection reports, clinical audit;
- feedback from supervisors; and
- outcomes from appraisal systems.

For front-line services this review should coincide with or precede any purchaser review so that the full position is understood internally before the external review takes place.

Summary

In this chapter possible measures were examined against the need to involve customers in defining those measures. Then phases in a systematic performance management plan were introduced, alongside possible appraisal systems. Finally, the need for review was highlighted.

References

Brinkerhoff, & Dressler (1990) *Productivity Measurement: A Guide for Managers and Evaluators.* Sage Publications, London.
Handy, C. (1994) *The Empty Raincoat: Making sense of the future.* Hutchison, London.
McGregor, D. (1960) *The Human Side of Enterprise.* McGraw-Hill, New York.

Chapter 9:
THE PERSONNEL
DEPARTMENT

Introduction

This book has so far stressed the primary role of managers in the personnel management task. What role exists then, if any, for a personnel department or for a specialist personnel officer? More importantly, how can managers get the best from that specialist resource if it exists? This chapter looks at personnel as a specialist set of activities and at the function's legitimacy in supporting health services management.

Consideration is first given to the range of roles which may exist for specialist personnel officers and the structures in which they may operate and then to what type of support managers may need in their task and how they can maximize the effectiveness of the support available to them. Finally, the future role for personnel specialists in the new health organization is outlined.

Learning outcomes

- To understand the roles, structure and organization of the personnel management function.

- To appreciate that managers have choices about the nature and source of their professional personnel support.

- To be able to recognize personnel strategy, policy and procedure and its effect on management practice.

Personnel manager and line manager conflict

Firstly, it is necessary to clarify the two organizational terms, 'line' and 'staff'. Line managers are those with overall responsibility for a defined department or unit and its operations. Line managers contribute directly to the provision of the service, be it patient care or support to care activities. Staff managers are people with particular professional expertise. They provide advice and services to the line or operational manager and are also involved in policy formation.

Personnel administration in relation to employees is a line management responsibility but a staff function. To help explain this paradox of terms, although personnel managers have specialist expertise, they have not got any direct authority. This is logical since ultimately the line managers will be held to account for the results achieved by their departments. The personnel specialist exists to give advice and guidance. If and how action is taken is ultimately a line management affair. Such an arrangement obviously offers endless opportunity for conflict and frustration.

Apart from this organizational aspect, other factors exist with potentiality for conflict. Staff managers tend on average to be younger or less experienced, and to have better formal education in management; they have different attitudes, styles of behaviour and vocabulary from typical line managers. Line managers on average tend to be older, to have worked up to management from one of the health professions but increasingly to have obtained an additional management qualification. Personnel managers have undergone expert training in a specific limited field. Conflict may arise because of different perceptions of the value of practical or vocational experience compared with education and training. Line or operational managers may often rightly doubt new ideas which are based solely on academic experience. The jargon shorthand used by both specialists and line managers may present a further barrier to the relationship.

A common cause of conflict arises from confusion between the personnel specialist and the line manager about responsibilities for staff management. Line managers might rely on their personnel support, who themselves believe the line manager is responsible, so both neglect the personnel agenda. Alternatively if the line manager and personnel specialist both believe they have prime responsibility for staff management in any area they will again conflict. The shades of orange are greater than the areas of red or yellow and so relative responsibilities are not obvious.

Personnel departments serve to provide top management with

information about different areas of the organization. This can breed suspicion and mistrust in line managers, and it may be considered (often justifiably) that staff managers have the ear of senior management. The nature of the specialism may also affect the situation. Although generally the reason for the existence of the staff functions is to help line managers achieve greater effectiveness and efficiency, some are more overtly involved in assessing and improving the line management than others and personnel can be seen as too interventionist.

With increasing legislation the personnel manager is forced to insist rather than advise. In this way, the personnel manager is having to intrude to an increasing degree into the special relationship that should exist between line managers and their staff. With some justification the line managers may consider their authority is being reduced.

The conflict is not, however, one-sided. The specialists may become equally embittered. They are likely to be frustrated by a lack of authority in instances where line managers do not request advice or worse refuse to accept it. Also, they may experience difficulties in line managers dismissing personnel management as a separate function warranting specialist skills. All managers see themselves managing their own personnel.

The next logical step is to seek resolution of this conflict. In general, there are no easy or short-term solutions. Senior management can give a lead by encouraging co-operation. Specialists should be constantly reminded that their role is to strengthen line management. The best situation is where personnel managers treat line managers as clients; to be given the best possible advice and then, where possible, allowed to accept or reject it. Alternative styles will be examined later in the chapter.

To a large extent, the success or otherwise of the specialist will be determined by personality and approach, whatever the organizational problems. Common objectives should be emphasized and problems tackled as a joint venture. The personnel specialist should always assess proposals in the light of the practical and real problems facing the line manager. Line managers are frequently overloaded with responsibilities directly linked to functional goals. Line managers are often, therefore, only too happy to pass non-operational aspects of their work on to a specialist.

Personnel's traditional purpose and structure

The task

Although differences obviously do exist, by sector and geography, traditional hospital and community personnel departments typically offer a range of administrative support services as described below:

(1) *Finding potential staff*

Writing job descriptions, personnel specifications and job advertisements, arranging interviews, administering selection tests, ensuring equality of opportunity, informing unsuccessful candidates and keeping records.

(2) *Employment of new staff*

Obtaining references, health screening, making the employment offer, determining a salary, preparing a contract, sending out joining instructions and arranging induction.

(3) *Maintaining structure*

Administering transfers and promotions, grading posts, keeping job descriptions, drawing and presenting structure charts and controlling the establishment.

(4) *Providing information*

Recording staff, personnel and post data, checking professional registrations, monitoring attendance levels, providing staff-in-post and vacancy data.

(5) *Communication*

Maintaining an information dissemination mechanism and systems for receiving employees' views, providing staff handbooks and other means of ensuring employees receive information about their employment.

(6) *Staff training*

Providing in-house courses, keeping information on external programmes, keeping educational and reference materials, booking staff on programmes.

(7) Health and welfare
> Arranging workplace safety audits, keeping accident statistics, administering a safety committee structure, administering staff redeployment.

(8) Managing the contractual relationship
> Providing advice on terms and conditions, advising on the grievance procedure, assisting in disciplinary matters.

(9) Managing leavers
> Ensuring dates and entitlements are met (be it resignation, maternity leave, dismissal or retirement), documenting the process, maintaining termination records, providing advice on preparation for retirement and statutory payments.

The typical duties described above are bound together by the postholder in an overriding professional philosophy described by Buckingham and Elliot (1993) as follows:

> 'This philosophy is strongly rooted in clear perceptions about, and real commitment to, the value of good employees and their contribution to the company.'

Managers may well decide that the kind of direct administrative support described above is what they need to relieve them of such chores. Putting the activities described all in one place allows the individual or department to make it their job and to become expert. It is easy to see how dealing with the above matters quickly becomes a busy and demanding role. Anyone responsible for fulfilling the role would start to have problems if the numbers of staff involved rose above about five hundred.

Some of the tasks described are hedged with legal constraints or duties, others will be covered by organizational policy and all by some sense of best practice. It is a simple step then to move the role described above from administrative support into guardianship of good procedure and practice. Allowing these roles to move in this way begins to create the 'line' and 'staff' conflict described earlier. Managers are allowed or not allowed to proceed in certain ways and have to consult the 'expert' personnel officer before acting. Accountability to ensure good personnel management then sits with the personnel officer rather than the manager. The primacy of the manager is lost.

This disadvantageous process can be avoided to some extent by giving careful thought to choices about the personnel officer's role. Lack of such role clarity also makes the personnel officer's role difficult. Managers may operate on a 'do not call me, I will call you' basis so that intervention is restricted. The major difficulty with this divorced arrangement is that the calls are only made when something has failed and so fire-fighting help is needed. Personnel officers object to being used as a rescue service when, with involvement earlier, they could have prevented problems. A decision has to be made whether to watch events go out of shape after a manager has not sought or ignored advice or to intervene with a more authoritative stance to avoid the later difficulties.

The roles

Staying with typical or traditional structures, presuming the organization concerned employs more than five hundred or so people then the personnel department will develop a set of roles in a hierarchy. These will have different local labels but typically can be characterized as follows.

(1) Personnel Assistant

Provides clerical and administrative support. This will include such items as sending out application forms, preparing and sending out contracts of employment, arranging interviews, maintaining files and records, providing instructions to the payroll section. Such posts may require a Certificate in Personnel Practice or similar.

(2) Personnel Officer

Provides professional support to managers in writing job descriptions, job advertisements and personnel specifications. Will attend and assist in selection interviews, grievance and disciplinary hearings, conduct maternity leave or retirement interviews and participate in a range of other direct staff management activities. Such posts may require a professional qualification e.g. graduate membership of the Institute of Personnel and Development.

(3) Personnel Manager

> Provides the procedural and policy framework and advice on that framework. Writes protocols for managers or personnel officers to follow across a range of personnel activities. Deals directly with more complex individual issues and with most collective staff interventions, such as restructuring or relocating a department. Such a person would have learnt employment law and best personnel practice which they can then apply to real life situations.

(4) Personnel Director/Head of Personnel

> Provides a direction for policy having monitored the outside environment and the needs of the organization. Providing advice to the Board on the human resources it needs and how those resources should be managed to best effect. For example, taking a view on the organization's stance towards formal employee relations having examined the amount of organizational change necessary of the next few years and the wider political context now and in the future. Such postholders also respond to national initiatives with Trust-wide policies i.e. on local pay bargaining.

Activity

Given the management task or specific problems that face you from a personnel standpoint which type of personnel role's time would help you the most at present:

Personnel Assistant	☐
Personnel Officer	☐
Personnel Manager	☐
Personnel Director	☐

Structure

So far this chapter has focused on the traditional or typical function. From here it will examine options for structure and roles. Some or all of the four roles described above may exist in health organizations. They may not, however, necessarily be seen in one department as a hierarchy of roles. Options exist for structuring the specialist human resources as shown below.

Central personnel departments

The traditional or typical structure is viewed as central and generalist as shown in Figure 9.1.

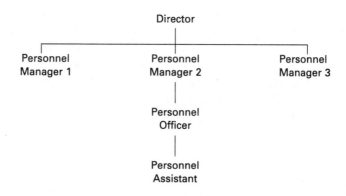

Fig. 9.1   Central generalist personnel structure.

Each personnel manager in the structure typically has a range of departments to whom they specifically offer a service. They can get to know the staff and managers in their 'patch' and so can provide relevant advice in context. Another possibility is that the central structure fragments into sub-specialisms of the personnel agenda as shown in Figure 9.2.

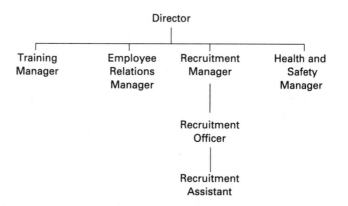

Fig. 9.2   Central specialist personnel structure.

In the instance above, the personnel managers in each branch are expert but do not relate specifically to any one part of the organization. Depth of technical expertise in a sub-specialism of personnel is gained at the cost of the managers being further removed from the various parts of the organization they are employed to serve.

To capitalize on the advantages of both possible configurations the central personnel managers may form a matrix structure. In such a structure personnel managers would have specific personnel service responsibilities to a range of departmental managers and at the same time have a specialist role across the organization. In Figure 9.1 Personnel Manager 1 would have special responsibility for training and so on.

However central structures are organized, they do have strengths and weaknesses.

Strengths

Centre of knowledge
Economy of scale
Centre of expertise
Potential for cover and support
Corporate focus
Unbiased

Weaknesses

Detached from care services
Inward looking
Professional rather than service agenda
Bureaucratic

Devolvement of the specialism

Central personnel departments suffer from the disadvantages listed above. It is also clear that personnel officers cannot contribute effectively unless they are close to and understand the business they are in. It is increasingly common to see central personnel departments in hospital and community Trusts divided into 'core' and 'operational' elements, with the operational element devolved to the line managers. The wider devolution and decentralization under way within the health sector is accelerating the wider trend of devolving personnel departments.

Core

The central core is normally small and concerned with the duties of the employer as a corporate entity. The role of the core is often defined as providing:

- strategic planning,
- professional support,
- organizational values,
- policy frameworks, and
- organizational structure.

Operational

Provision of services in operational units of the organization is the role of the devolved sub-divisions of the personnel resource. Devolved personnel staff often have their managerial account-ability to their line manager and a professional line of accountability to the personnel core. Devolved specialists can make an integrated contribution as a member of the mainstream service management team. The focus of their contribution and loyalty is clear and to the manager they serve. This structure is illustrated in Figure 9.3.

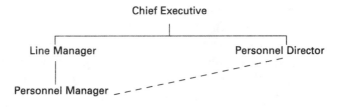

Fig. 9.3 Devolved personnel structure.

Devolvement to managers

If a specialist resource is hard to justify in a cost conscious organization then line managers can take on day-to-day per-sonnel activities given the skills they need to do the job com-petently. Line managers can often resist additional work unless they can also see the benefits of taking that work on. Simply 'dumping' onto managers the personnel administration which they used to have support for will not be welcomed. Giving managers the freedoms associated with disinvesting the struc-ture of a controlling personnel bureaucracy can, however, be attractive. While managers may be keen to obtain that freedom they will wish to be equipped and competent to exercise their own judgment. Managers do not want to become fully fledged expert personnel managers but it is not surprising to find that experienced managers know more about personnel management than they or the personnel department realize.

To achieve a successful devolution of personnel to the line the organization needs to be clear about its definition of 'personnel' and what it is requiring managers to do for themselves. Managers need to be clear about what support they need to allow then to operate their own staff management. How much of the existing personnel resource can be released depends on the work transferred and the support required to sustain it.

A risk assessment is also a sensible to establish the likely effect of removing or managing without personnel specialists, in the short and medium term.

Outsourcing

In other parts of the public sector personnel activities viewed as non-core, such as recruitment administration, are being outsourced. Personnel departments, if they exist in-house, have to devolve their budgets and it is then up to the managers as customers whether or not they choose to buy back the service. Organizations need to be prepared to devolve budgets to allow such outsourcing. If the service is purchased by line managers then they may not source it from the traditional providers. Competitive tendering can equally apply to staff services such as personnel support. Smaller organizations which cannot afford to employ personnel expertise directly have no option but to obtain outside advice as and when they require it.

'Customer' is a difficult term for personnel officers as it may be that prospective employees, existing employees, line managers or the employing organization are all customers. The needs of these groups may differ if not conflict. Handing the purse strings (and so the decision to buy services) to individual line managers makes their primacy explicit, as, to a lesser extent, does having the employer competitively test the service. Treating personnel specialists as a sub-contractors may increase value for money against pre-defined services but it removes a source of expertise from the business so that it is neither as integral nor as flexible. An internal department must be allowed to compete for the provision of services outside the host organization if internal managers are allowed to source their services from outside.

If money follows customer satisfaction then internal personnel standards will be even more difficult to enforce. The customer is always right – even if they are wrong!

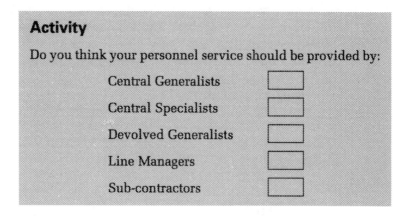

Activity

Do you think your personnel service should be provided by:

Central Generalists

Central Specialists

Devolved Generalists

Line Managers

Sub-contractors

Service level agreements

If the existing service is important or is not providing satisfaction then a service level agreement may help to ensure reliability.

However if the existing service is structurally organized, it is possible to put in place a service level agreement, possibly as a first step toward market testing but more likely as a means of clarifying expectations. If the service continues to fail to meet managers' needs under such an agreement then it is possible to seek alterations. A service level agreement is usually:

- written,
- agreed between user and provider,
- a service definition, and
- a statement of standards.

Managers may wish to define:

- the specification of services provided,
- response times and work schedules,
- the quality of service,

- activity levels, and
- charges.

Such an agreement will facilitate a closer relationship between the personnel service and its users. The disadvantage is that such agreements tend to focus on specific short-term internal standards, such as responding to job enquiries within 12 hours, missing the longer term targets which require an integrated approach between managers and personnel such as labour turnover, absence levels or unit labour costs. If line managers spend half an hour together with the question 'What do you require from your personnel department?' the flip-chart typically looks like the one in Figure 9.4.

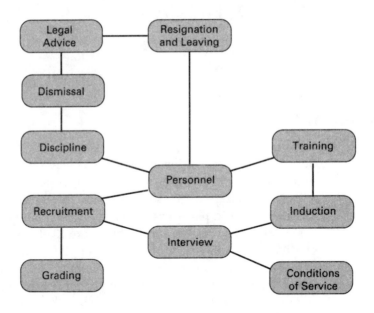

Fig. 9.4 Personnel's role – a manager's view.

The danger of leaving a service provided to managers to be defined through demand is that they can have a very limited view of what they want or need. The exclusions from the output above might be because of positive choices, accidental omission or ignorance arising from a lack of experience of requiring support.

Styles of personnel management

The dominant value systems within the personnel profession have changed over the century reflecting the values and problems of the time. In brief summary they can be characterized as follows.

(1) *Moral crusader (concerned with charity)*

In the early 1900s welfare officers were retained by employers or provided by charities to help alleviate the poor conditions of industrial workers. These welfare officers, if employed, supplemented the work of the charitable and welfare organizations. Sympathies or motives lay alongside the beginnings of the trade union movement.

(2) *Employee advocate (concerned with well-being)*

Social and behavioural studies in the 1930s and 1940s caused employers to think again about workers and their importance to future successful business enterprise. The concept of the happy, motivated, productive worker was born and personnel professionals, from a social science base, sought to create such workers through manipulation of human relationships.

(3) *Management advocate (concerned with control)*

In the 1960s and 1970s the power of the trade unions was high and their influence increasing. Personnel officers were representatives of management in the collective bargaining arena and often found themselves in conflict with staff interests.

(4) *Law enforcer (concerned with compliance)*

Throughout the 1970s and 1980s Parliament passed a huge amount of new employment legislation. It fell to the personnel function as 'experts' to see that law implemented in the workplace and to see that managers acted in compliance with the statutory requirements concerning employment.

(5) *Economist (concerned with efficiency)*

The 1980s and 1990s meant recession and a new political ideology so that management saw staff as an economic resource and 'personnel' as the people to ensure its best utilization in the workplace. It was during this time that human resource management became an advanced concept.

An element of each of these very broad descriptions still, each in their own way, stays with the profession adding to its richness and diversity. As Derek Torrington (1989) said, 'Personnel management has grown through the assimilation of a number of different emphases to produce an ever-richer combination of expertise'. Managers may, however, want to establish from their own personnel advice source which value base it primarily operates from. A feeling persists amongst managers and employees that personnel practitioners are in some way neutral and so more likely to exercise judgment with fairness and equity in mind. However, it is difficult to be impartial when one side pays the salary! Another myth, which again has little foundation, seems to be that personnel is the moral or ethical face of management.

Behavioural category of personnel intervention

Managers can now have choices in the style of their personnel service. The choices broadly are to have a service which is provided by:

- a manager,
- a consultant,
- a coach, or
- an adviser.

Personnel manager

Personnel managers have executive authority to intervene where they see a need and to act, with the line manager where possible, to gain the outcomes sought. Personnel managers can ensure that managers follow certain policies or procedures and can monitor practice to ensure compliance. Line managers faced with a staff problem are sure to accept the attention and instruction of the personnel manager to ensure the best possible outcome.

Personnel consultant

Consultants come into a service once their entry has been requested, normally for a specific and defined purpose. A brief is given to the consultant who then carries out the work as an assignment, perhaps providing recommendations. The manager is free to accept or reject the 'proposal for work' or any resulting recommendations or advice. If a consultant comes across other problems or concerns while conducting one assignment no remit to act exists without a fresh mandate.

Personnel coach

The coach looks to assist those managers who need support and guidance. The coach allows managers to shape their own objectives and progress, doing as much or as little as each manager's own competence in each situation demands. The aim of such coaches is to work themselves out of their jobs by ensuring, through a process of personal development, that managers can act independently in all circumstances.

Personnel adviser

The adviser is an expert who, given information about the situation facing the manager, can provide a range of possible solutions based on best practice or a specific answer. The adviser takes no direct action to assist the manager to proceed in a more informed way. The adviser often has no vested interest in ensuring that managers are successful in their endeavours but is concerned that the advice the managers get is good advice.

The style of service the manager gets may depend on the culture of the organization, the mission of the personnel organization or the people in post. Rather than allowing the style adopted to be a happy (or unhappy) accident some explicit debate among the managers may be helpful to clarify their expectations. Some personnel practitioners can change their style to suit, but some are not capable of a transition between the types described above. Personnel specialists need to be engaged in the debate about the level, place and style of their support so that there is a clear consent.

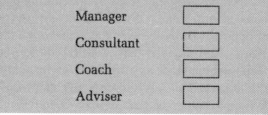

Activity

Which style of personnel practitioner would you be most comfortable with receiving your services from:

Manager ☐

Consultant ☐

Coach ☐

Adviser ☐

Orientation

Two orientations presently battle it out intellectually for centre stage. The contenders are personnel management and human resource management. Many outsiders are left asking whether or not a difference exists, whether one just reflects the Americanization of our language rather than a different orientation. However, the two are different and the supporters of the one concept do not support the other. One wishes to 'put the people back into personnel' while the other faces the new reality of competitive product and labour markets.

(1) Personnel management

The traditional staff officer or personnel professional carries a strong belief in the important place of people at work – their relationships and the ways to motivate them to give their best. In the eyes of the traditional personnel manager well managed employees and good employers operating best employment practices make a winning combination. They are characterized by people orientated values, a focus on people's strengths and a strong sense of business ethics. This may express itself in a view of personnel as an arbiter for or between staff and management, as a friend of both aiming to maintain their relationship and meet their needs. Buckingham (1993) says:

> 'They have gifts of insight in understanding how a person could develop, what kind of innate strengths they could call on, and which kind of experiences, opportunities, and team combinations might enable them to really blossom and become the best they can be.'

(2) Human resource management

The new orientation is concerned primarily with getting the best return from people at work by integrating people and business management. Human resource managers see people as a cost, or more positively as an investment, on which the business seeks a return. They believe that it is the appropriate investment in people which gives any organization its competitive advantage over others. The key difference is expressed by Hendry and Pettigrew (1986) in that human resource managers maintain 'there is no reason in principle why an employment strategy has to be employee centred'.

It is not always, but sometimes, the best employment practice which prevails, but the answer lies in the best fit between the two orientations.

Personnel framework

Strategy, policy and procedure

Personnel departments will draw up written documents which will be classified as either strategy, policy or procedure. Each has a very different purpose and each is explored below with examples given.

Personnel strategy

Strategy in the personnel context cannot exist of its own, it has to relate employment to

- the business as it is now and in the future,
- the wider environment including the state of the labour market,
- government policy, and
- the health economy.

The personnel strategy may not be distinct from the organization's overall statement of strategic directions; certainly the two cannot be divorced. The strategy will address

- the numbers of staff required,
- the type of organization and structure required,
- necessary values,
- changes in skills demanded,
- competition expected, and
- the factors for future success.

To determine the future of employment in the organization the predicted future of the organization is required. Personnel strategy does not just react to the business strategy but also it informs that wider strategy in terms of feasibility and possibilities. Is the organization seeking:

- to expand into new areas or retrench?
- to sell on the basis of quality or value for money?
- to invest in new technology?

Each business decision has a direct impact on employment.

Policy

Personnel policies are expressions of the organization's decisions, for each aspect of employment, made in the context of the
overall direction. The policy framework assists managers and
personnel managers operate by broadly directing their actions.
By following policy, managers should know that they are
operating with authority and within the law, making decisions
consistent with those made by other managers and appropriate
to the organization's longer-term wishes. Policies may exist on a
range of matters including:

- training and development,
- management development,
- health and safety,
- managing ill-health,
- managing incapability,
- managing misconduct,
- reward,
- recruitment, and so on.

Procedure

Procedures are detailed step-by-step guides setting out how to
conduct a particular operation so that managers are guided as to
how to proceed in their day-to-day work.

To take a couple of examples, firstly, the personnel strategy
might suggest that people should be rewarded for the responsibility they carry and the contribution they make. A reward
policy may then follow on with those strategic intentions
through job evaluation and performance related pay. The procedure would tell managers how to get a job graded or how to
conduct an appraisal. Secondly, the personnel strategy may
suggest that everyone should be developed to their full potential. The policy would then perhaps introduce training needs
analysis and development centres. A procedure would instruct
managers how to purchase or book training.

Given the above arrangements, managers could not pay
people on the basis of age, service or friendship, nor could
they develop people to only the minimum job requirement.
Alternative strategies could have made these possible
behaviours.

Bureaucracy

Some organizations adopt very detailed sets of policy and procedure so that managers have to obtain a detailed knowledge of the rules and follow them. In such organizations good management is expressed as the ability to select appropriately and adhere to the correct routine for each situation that arises. Many health service organizations are like this, with managers having access to manuals on topics such as Management Policy and Procedure, Personnel Policy and Procedure, a Health and Safety Manual, a Finance Manual, a Patient Care and Quality Manual, and so on. This is in addition to a detailed set of employee terms and conditions. The justification for such paper based control is that health services are complex organizations and managers cannot know everything, so regulation provides a security of practice. The danger is that managers get lost in the forest in the search for the right tree to climb. If a situation is not covered by a protocol then inaction results until instructions are provided.

Other organizations manage through a set of statements of core values which act to guide managers on their own decision-making. Rather than looking for a procedure, the managers have to consider for themselves the events ahead of them and decide what to do guided by stated values or desired outcomes. The advantages are that managers can be innovative, they can act to solve their own problems as they see fit, and are not tightly constrained. The disadvantage is that managers in such environments have to give problems greater attention and they refer more to senior managers as processes are not automatic. Freedom is time consuming, can create inconsistencies and insecurity and is a risk to the organization.

Summary

This chapter examined the difference between personnel and line managers and the roles personnel specialists fulfil. It went on to look at the organization of personnel specialists, their values and the different styles adopted. Finally, the place of strategies, policies and procedures was shown.

Recommended further reading

Consider T. Plant (1993) Occasional Paper No 4. *The Role of Clinical Directorates in Pay and Personnel Decisions*, and the piece by D. Guest and R. Peccei (1992), *The effectiveness of Personnel Management in the NHS* which was compiled as a result of research undertaken on behalf of the Department of Health.

References

Buckingham, G. & Elliot, G. (1993). Profile of a successful personnel manager. *Personnel Management.*

Hendry, C. & Pettigrew, A. (1986) The Practice of Human Resource Management. *Personnel Review* **15** (5), 3–8.

Torrington, D. (1989) Human Resource Management and the Personnel Function? In *New Perspectives on Human Resource Management.* Routledge, London.

Further Information

Institute of Personnel and Development
IPD House
Camp Road
Wimbledon
London
SW19 4UX
Tel. 0181 971 9000
Fax. 0181 263 3333

Chapter 10:
A LOOK FORWARD

Introduction

It is often prudent to look ahead and to take a view on what organizational and operational developments are likely to take place. In observing the future for hospital staff and staff management it is necessary first to see the wider picture. The health service is subject to both political and policy decisions so it may be considered that any view of the future is likely to be filled with uncertainty. However, although uncertainty does exist, certain facts do remain constant regardless of the political colour of the government or the shape of NHS Executive policy. These realities and their inevitable consequences follow the trends in health care and the possible future based on those trends. The focus of this chapter will be on the impact of the predicted future on employment patterns and the consequences for staff management.

Learning outcomes

- To gain an appreciation of the trends in health care delivery and the impact of those trends on health institutions.

- To gain an appreciation of the broad employment trends in the UK and the impact of those trends on health service employment.

- To perceive the consequences of both the above for managers, personnel managers and staff in the health sector.

Broad health trends

The first stage of this analysis of the likely future is to describe what is happening in health.

Non-political factors

In macro terms there are the non-political factors considered below.

Demand

As public education about health improves so demands placed on the health care system will increase. People will expect more care and better quality care than previous generations. The increasing age and related dependency of the population will accelerate this growing demand or expectation.

Standards

Attitudes toward public services have become more critical and demanding. The Patient's Charter and performance tables are the current expressions of increasing expectations and the standards sought will probably rise.

Treatments

Improvements in medicine and the development of new treatments will extend the range of possible services and so decisions about what should be available free from the NHS will become more difficult. However, techniques such as endoscopy promise to revolutionize treatment times and surgical productivity. Nevertheless, some sections of the population will need or be required to make their own provisions for health care, as highlighted by the move of some elderly care to Social Services so introducing means testing and payment. Non-treatment of smokers for certain conditions related to smoking is sometimes raised.

Localization

People will increasingly, if not predominantly, be treated on a day-care basis; in their homes or in general practitioner-led facilities. As the trend to treat more people outside of hospitals continues so the number of hospital beds will continue to fall as has been happening since 1948.

Changing institutions

The changes described in the nature of the population and the care which that population demands will have an impact on the current institutions. Broadly, the changes can be perceived and described for purchasers and providers as shown below.

Purchasers

At present District Health Authorities or Commissions and general practitioners purchase care. The roles of those two purchasing groups will become distinct and diverse. As acute care provision covers larger geographical catchment areas, the number of potential providers increases and transfer between them becomes more critical, so commissioning will widen both in scope and geography. At the local level leadership will come from general practitioners within their localities who will provide more care themselves and will inform the secondary and tertiary care providers of their communities' needs.

In 1994 the Secretary of State published a paper, *Developing NHS Purchasing and GP Fundholding: Toward a Primary Care-Led NHS* which expanded the role of fundholding general practitioners. The accompanying letter EL(94)79 stated that there would be three types of fundholding:

- community fundholding,
- standard fundholding,
- total purchasing.

While fundholding of itself may not survive political change the involvement of general practitioners in service provision which it represents is likely to continue.

Providers

The mix of providers will change and the number of players in that new mix will increase as the pattern of service delivery shifts. Social services, voluntary organizations, private organizations and community NHS Trusts will all look to provide holistic care as the acute sector moves to minimum intensive intervention.

Community Hospitals have suffered since the early 1960s with the introduction of District General Hospitals. However, as the number of procedures that can be undertaken on an outpatient or day-case basis are increased, so work will be undertaken in the patient's locality rather than in large city hospitals. General practitioners will take up much of the provision for minor acute and diagnostic work, possibly extending their range through locally purchased consultant-led sessions in community hospitals. The shorter lengths of acute hospital stays will require a more sophisticated short-term/post-operative level of care than currently provided. Community hospitals may flourish again.

'Care in the community', shifts to practice-centred primary care (and secondary care outside of hospitals), falling bed numbers, expansion of day surgery; shorter lengths of stay, 'hospital at home' and expanded community hospitals will each decrease the need for general hospital capacity. The number of hospitals will continue to fall as they close or merge. Paradoxically, the more intensive specialized nature of the acute care which remains means it has to take place in a smaller number of 'super' hospitals and will increase the cost per case.

Political dynamic

There is a specifically political complexion to the above in that the Conservative Government which introduced the 1990 legislation believed the changes would be best achieved through competition within a managed market. The active encouragement of alternative private providers of care or sources of funds would, it was thought, add to the level of competition and allow state involvement to be rolled back. NHS Trusts and general practitioner fundholding, being created by legislation, could be dismantled by future legislation, but the changes listed above are, as has been seen, not driven by those labels. They emerged from social and technological factors, although that emergence was facilitated by politics.

The existing community and acute hospitals, their Boards, employees and surrounding communities will not want their institutions to close or to merge with other hospitals in nearby towns on cities. The wish of each of the present 300 or so Trusts will be to survive in the internal market. This instinct will cause Trust Boards to drive down cost per case prices, increase throughput of patients and promote the quality of their care. Boards will be defensive of their existing local services and, with increasing aggression, will seek to expand the populations they serve. The fact is that they cannot all be successful. In the shake-out that is to come each will fight to be the survivor whether or not that is logical or desirable from a wider planned perspective. A few will grow into regional centres, many more will become smaller and a few will merge or close. Trust Boards in their strategic directions will need to decide whether withdrawal from certain services or localities is an option and whether such withdrawal will be through choice or competitive forces.

Trust Boards and their service managers need to identify:

- core facilities necessary for future viability,
- key services which should be maintained and defended, and
- services which could be lost, however unfortunate.

Further, in the light of that analysis managers should:

- plan for disinvestment,
- develop marketing plans based on their strengths, and
- seek to expand or underpin key services.

Purchasers could put some planned sense of direction into the market by making appropriate longer-term commitments to providers who have a future role in the partnership. Providers will find it difficult to plan to expand or shrink without a guaranteed level of funding, indicating a need for longer-term rolling contracts rather than annual ones. Clear direction from purchasers would help providers to decide whether or not to compete.

Broad employment trends

Having examined the part of the picture related to health services the second part is employment generally in the UK.

General trends

Again, in broad terms the factors are as follows.

Demography

Despite economic recession hiding the short-term effects, underlying population changes remain which will reduce the number of people available for work and particularly the number of young people. The supply of potential traditional entrants into the health professions will tighten.

Employment

The structure of employment, that is the types of jobs available (and the nature of those jobs) will change. Overall there will be an increase in jobs but inside this overall growth some sectors including manufacturing will continue to see large scale labour reductions.

Education

Education is becoming increasingly vocational, that is training people in skills for jobs. Competence will become more important than knowledge. Given the demographic and employment changes much education will be re-training for new areas of work where shortages will exist. This is characterized by the recent merger of the Employment Department into the Department for Education.

Social protection

European social policy will have a continued and increasing effect on the UK despite current attempts to restrict some elements which place a financial burden on employers. The setting of minimum standards will put in place a baseline wage below which it will be illegal to employ anyone but above which may be simply uneconomic to do so. As UK labour is currently relatively inexpensive, it is argued that any attempt to equalize across Europe will be at the cost of local employers and jobs.

Social values

The role of women at work across a range of jobs and sectors will continue to expand. The potential for the participation of women at work combined with demographically caused staff shortages will place increased pressure on both government and employers for family-friendly policies. The number of part-time jobs or job-shares will increase in the growth areas of the economy.

Management development

While formal management education is a more recent development in the UK than elsewhere, significant improvements in the development and education of British managers will continue alongside the trend to see increasing integration across the management disciplines. Functional specialism will continue to decline in value in the eyes of employers.

Mobility

From the development of the railways in the middle of the last century to Norman Tebbit's exhortation to 'get on your bike', the trend has been towards increasing mobility of the labour force. However, continued differentials in house prices and the cost of living between regions, combined with (in the short term) a dramatic fall in property prices and 'negative equity', militate against labour movement. Moreover, the increasing number of families with dual careers also has an effect on the individual decision-making surrounding relocation. Given these factors, the presumption that some posts have a national catchment population may be false.

Health service employment

The environment described above for health and employment allows a generalized view to develop about the future of employment in health services. By making predictions about employment, the consequences for health service managers can be observed in their personnel management role.

Service delivery

High skill levels will be drawn to or concentrated in the specialist regional centres. In general the health service will see a reduction in professionalism which will be replaced in part by a more vocational and competent workforce. This replacement workforce will predominantly be client or population focused rather than focused on a particular institution or building.

Work categories

Head-count reductions and competitive pressure will demand flexibility between the roles of health workers. Changing contractual demands from purchasers will require adaptability and increased multi-skilling of employees and their organizations if both are to survive the turbulence ahead.

Employment

The number of potential employers in any particular market will increase in the short term preceding a shake-out caused by competitive pressure. Employees will either through choice, competitive tendering or take-over find their employers changing as the traditional steady state comes to an end.

If the employer chooses or is forced to withdraw from service provision in a given area, some employees may find that they are redundant. The service provision may relocate between hospitals or agencies, or from existing service providers to new. Managers will not be able to offer substantive permanent positions or promise only to introduce changes to work with understanding and agreement. If their employment base is to have any security then individuals will need to be flexible and must expect and accept change.

Wages

In order to retain business in a market which differentiates between providers on price and given local pay flexibility employers will look to reduce unit labour costs to stay competitive. However, within this generalization, certain key staff in short supply may demand additional pay or privileges which the more successful providers will be able to afford.

If local pay determination does not exist then national rates apply and pay may be more of a level playing field and so quality, productivity and pay costs (i.e. differences in numbers, grades and skill-mix) will prevail. Again, the survivors will be those who can keep overall costs down while retaining key skills.

Consequences for managers

The first and most obvious consequence of all the above for health service managers is that they are approaching an uncharted period of change and uncertainty in health provision. Health service staff are not used to real change in service but are used to structural re-organization. While the reforms represented a significant cultural change within health services the effects of those changes will be even more dramatic. In London (and other areas where there is a perceived over-provision of acute service for the local population) the cold winds of the now more than notional 'internal' market are already being felt. While London is the subject of some central planning, elsewhere general practitioners will create a pace of change through fundholding that will not be planned in the traditional sense.

Service closure and job losses will not be rational or planned within the organization where staff can challenge the choices made, but change will be the ultimate consequence of internal decision-making.

At the same time managers will need to undertake a strategic analysis to anticipate the future for their particular service. They will, within the surrounding uncertainty, need to ensure the survival and success of their service – or its planned demise if that is inevitable given the strategic analysis. Some of the changes that may be required to ensure survival and future success may place a particular manager in conflict with professional idealism or traditional notions of fairness or equity. Individual managers will then have to decide whether their loyalty is to themselves, their profession, their employer or to the patients or clients.

For example, a host purchaser may buy an inpatient service with a quality standard that patients should wait no longer than one year, a neighbouring purchaser may purchase with a standard of nine months, and local fundholders may buy on the basis of a waiting time of six months. The manager may be keen to attract these alternative purchasers and to foster a good relationship with them. The clinical staff, however, will have difficulty juggling the individual quality standards set out in the different contracts. The manager will have to negotiate with clinical staff within the organization to accept the purchasers' different standards, because retaining their custom may make the difference between viability and difficulty.

To take another example, doctors see themselves in many respects as private practitioners as well as employees of a particular NHS institution. A doctor might, therefore, be approached by a fundholding general practitioner to undertake work as a private individual outside the NHS contract. The fact that the same work was destined for the Trust and so represents lost revenue to the service that employs the doctor may not register, or if it does it may not seem relevant to the individual concerned.

Perhaps the last relevant illustration to complete this picture is of professional defensiveness. A scattering of senior professionals reject attempts by managers to start a constructive dialogue about skill-mix, the introduction of trained support workers on wards, departments or into localities to assist the registered professionals with their duties through appropriate delegation. Such approaches are often seen as an overt threat to the profession, going against the principles of primary nursing which essentially suggest that the registered professional, however expensive, should do everything. Even when clinical services are under threat of competitive tendering and the service is known to be relatively expensive (primarily because of staff costs) such professional resistance tends to persist.

If managers have to negotiate externally with purchasers and internally with staff in a contractual environment of uncertainty, then, when the staff do not perceive where their best long-term interest may lie, patience and persistence will be needed! Devolved accountability and the internal market put pressure on decision makers to develop a focus on the employer rather than a corporate NHS or professional focus. In that insular sense the manager needs to do whatever it takes to achieve business objectives although that may sometimes be in the face of internal opposition. If the professional ethic to provide best quality care gives way to market forces then this raises the question of whether ethical values have a place in today's health care. Managers will not fail to observe standing orders or standing financial instructions so clearly minimum standards do apply. Equally, abusing a public position for personal gain is not acceptable. It is difficult to ask managers to act in an impartial way when they have a clear interest in the survival of their organization, whether or not it is actually needed to treat and care for patients or clients into the future. Managers in public service do, however, need to act responsibly and with integrity.

Public service or professional values are not necessarily suffering within a system of devolved management and local accountability. Those values do, however, need redefining over time so that they are relevant and constant within the contemporary environment. It is not enough to suggest that ethics is a matter for an individual's private soul; the behaviour of public servants is a matter of public account.

Consequences for the personnel function

At organization level the personnel function should assess the demands and constraints facing the organization and develop resourcing plans. Clear plans would help managers to avoid short-term expedient staff changes in reaction to market situations which unnecessarily disrupt peoples lives.

To achieve this the great majority of personnel administration and activities should be passed back to line managers. Personnel roles which exist solely to act as hand maidens or surrogate managers should be abolished. The remaining small core of specialist personnel expertise would then be concerned with strategic human resource management, overseeing broad personnel policy issues.

Pressure on management costs, the limits on executive board members, the move away from functional specialism and the demise of trade unions each serve to make it less likely that a head of personnel will hold board level director status. The current change from national to local pay determination may act to reserve a place for senior personnel specialists on the Board but this is not sustainable beyond the short term. A Labour government and introduction of the Social Chapter may provide another issue to maintain the status of the specialist functional head.

The personnel agenda needs to change within health provision in response to either a removal of the internal market or a shake-out of weaker participants within that market. Cutting costs and making the survivors work harder is not a policy which can be sustained. Once NHS Trusts have cut staff costs to get themselves out of market difficulties and have established a firm customer base then a positive agenda must be introduced. Employee commitment and motivation, a will to have the Trust succeed, is not born from a fear of redundancy.

Consequences for staff

Clearly if organizations are to make the necessary changes and succeed they need the loyalty of their staff. Trusts and their Boards are new enough that demanding such loyalty may be premature in the view of staff interests. Staff organizations in the health service often act as both trade union and professional association, causing members to sometimes confuse self-interest, professional interest and patient interest as the conflicting messages they receive come from a single representative organization. These organizations often do have staff loyalty and so they may increasingly find in the short term that they are in conflict with NHS Trusts.

Individual employees will need to look to continuous professional development so as to maintain their employability in a difficult and changing environment. There is no longer an obvious progression in a single organization or the prospect of long-term employment.

Summary

This chapter has examined broad trends in health, politics and employment. Following this analysis, the consequences for employment in the health services are identified, followed by comments specifically related to managers, personnel specialists and staff. This non-specific look across the generality of health trends shows that managers need to look at their own local context, including local purchasing intentions and the local providers' business plans.

This book clearly suggests that managers, in looking at their own services and what the future holds, take account of and are informed by their service's human resources capability. Staff numbers, costs, skills and productivity will clearly make a difference. Staff, the skills they hold and the quality of service they provide are inseparable. These factors can be managed to best advantage but not by personnel specialists.

Reference

Bottomley, V. (Secretary of State for Health) (1994) EL(94)79. *Developing NHS purchasing and GP fundholding: Towards a Primary Care-led NHS*. NHS Executive, Department of Health.

INDEX

vacancy scrutiny, 22–3

wages, 13
waiting lists, 2
Weber, M., 63

Whitley Council, 12, 98, 100–
    102, 106, 110
workforce plans, 48–52
Working for Patients, 98